# Infertility

## A Survival Guide for Couples and Those Who Love Them

♥

Cindy Lewis Dake

New Hope Publishers
Birmingham, Alabama

New Hope Publishers
P. O. Box 12065
Birmingham, AL 35202-2065
www.newhopepubl.com

Cover design by Righteous Planet Design Studio, Franklin, Tennessee

ISBN: 1-56309-730-3
N024105•0102•5MI

♥

# For Edward

*For the million ways you helped,
advised, supported, comforted,
encouraged, and contributed.
—Thank you.*

*and*

# For Ryan

*Your arrival in our lives
didn't end our infertility.
But your presence makes its burden
so much easier to bear.
Your smile and laughter
light up our lives.
We love you so.*

♥

# Contents

# *Foreword*

Having been in the ministry for approximately 50 years, I have had my share of opportunities to share in the sorrows and losses of others. Most obvious is the loss of a loved one in the form of death. This brings about a painful grieving process that most adults are familiar with in one way or another. This grief, though painful, is usually accompanied by support from others, especially those who understand the pain firsthand. It is also a grief that, thankfully, tends to diminish over time as we adjust to the loss.

But there is another grief that is quite different. It is not experienced as widely nor understood as deeply as other kinds of grief. It is infertility—the subject of this book. Perhaps because infertility is so painful and carries such a sense of personal failure, most remain quiet about it. But let's understand one thing, it is a loss. It is the loss of feeling a sense of control. More personally, it is the loss of a dream. It can feel like the loss of one's sexual identity. We don't write obituaries for miscarriages, but the private feeling of abandonment by God and aloneness in a family-oriented world can be overwhelming at times. The poet has said that no man is an island, but that doesn't mean we don't feel like one at times.

This profound feeling of isolation can most effectively be bridged by one who has been there. Cindy Dake—along with her husband, Edward—clearly possesses the tools and experience to build such a bridge. (There is a chapter to men written by Edward). Not only does she know the island well, but Cindy also knows how to blend her personal experience with that of others, how to research thoroughly, and how to write in a friendly, candid style that brings it all right into your heart. As helpful as all that is, there is something else that sets this work apart from just another fellow traveler's story. It is the personal depth of the writer. I know the reader will appreciate the emotional and spiritual maturity Cindy brings to her understanding of infertility.

In addition to powerful testimonies representing the wide range of experiences, perhaps Cindy's greatest contribution is a biblical and theological perspective to address the many questions that arise in the lives of those battling infertility. These questions range from dealing with guilt, shame, victimization, and self-image to bargaining with God for "favorable treatment." Cindy deals with these questions in a refreshingly honest manner, while staying grounded in the Word and sensitive to the tender feelings of the reader.

This strength is built into the foundation of the many practical insights and concrete suggestions found from cover to cover. Cindy has included wise and wonderful tips for handling everything from insensitive comments by friends and family to setting boundaries for time and money invested in various child-bearing options.

Finally, let me applaud the inclusion of the option of adoption. While adoption may not be right for all infertile couples, it is a blessing to many parents and children. Once again, Cindy has earned the right to be heard on this subject as the reader quickly discovers. She also recognizes that, for some others, the acceptance of a childfree choice can bring its own unique blessings.

For years, as both a seminary professor and now as a pastor, I have emphasized the power of members of the body of Christ to minister to one another. I believe this book is one great example of this power in action. The silent pain of the infertile couple has produced a voice that resonates with those who are worthy to be heard. If you are struggling with infertility or know someone who is, be grateful for the labor of love represented in this work. Read it and be an instrument of God's love to others.

Dr. Gene A. Getz
Sr. Pastor, Fellowship Bible Church North
Director, Center for Church Renewal
Host and Teacher, Renewal Radio
Plano, TX

# Preface

When New Hope Publishers approached me about writing a book on infertility, I immediately was drawn to the topic of *surviving* infertility. Through our journey, Edward and I have learned that infertility can destroy us if we let it. But if we resolutely set ourselves to survive it, we can, with the love and support of family and friends and the strength and provision of our loving Father in heaven.

Survival isn't synonymous with success, by the way. If you measure success in terms of beating infertility by finally birthing a baby, then I'm a failure. But I sure don't feel like a failure. I have been blessed. I am a survivor who is glad to reach out to help others who are trekking through the valley.

## What you'll find in this book

Help for yourself; and guidance for helping others: that's it in a nutshell. This book is written primarily for the couple trying to navigate the confusing terrain of the "Valley of Infertility." For the person who wants to encourage an infertile friend, every chapter doubles as a how-to-understand-what-they're-going-through guide. On behalf of all of us who have struggled with infertility, thanks in advance for caring enough to read about what we're going through.

Woven throughout the chapters are quotes from others who have battled infertility. I am intrigued by the wisdom of those who have shared their infertility journeys with me. Their actual words let you glimpse into their lives and their journey.

Infertile couples need to know that they are not alone. A couple can feel absolutely alone in infertility because their journey is unlike anyone else's. Eventually, you will begin to look around and see that other people have been through it; but for a while you can only see your own battle. This book is packed with stories of other couples' infertility experiences. I interviewed about thirty infertile couples in person, on the phone, and via email. Some have birthed a child, others have adopted, and some have chosen not to continue pursuing children of their own. One couple's marriage didn't survive. Their stories will captivate you.

Resources for further study are included at the end of the book. I had a choice: Include a plethora of book titles to give you an overwhelming selection or include a short list of titles based on my personal experience with them. I opted for the latter: A long list of books can be immobilizing for someone bearing the grief of infertility.

The same goes for Web sites. The problem with publishing Internet addresses is the transitory nature of Web life. A site can be up today and lost in cyberspace tomorrow. I have listed only the very best sites I could find—ones that are part of organizations that will be around for a long time. To find smaller sites hosted by everyday people—and these sites have definite merit—just search the Internet by topic, such as Neonatal Death, Child-free Living, etc.

### Those who have helped me survive

Surviving infertility was one thing; surviving this book was quite another! I don't have adequate words to thank my husband, Edward, who has helped me research practically every aspect of this book. Edward can find anything on the Internet in record time. He wrote the chapter "A Man's Perspective on Infertility," and read, reviewed, and commented on the others. Besides that, he spent many evenings entertaining Ryan so I could handcuff myself to the computer. He has picked up dinners to go, pulled more than his share of the household chores, and has sacrificed his time in so many ways.

My mom, Sandra Lewis, deserves a huge thank-you. She gave round-the-clock care to Ryan for at least fifty days in five months, not to mention the laundry and dishes she's washed for us along the way. She gave up her own schedule and ministry activities, and put her life on hold so that I could push forward. This book wouldn't have been finished by deadline without her.

I'm also grateful to my mother-in-law, Sandra Davis, and my sister-in-law, Amy Lewis, who watched Ryan on several occasions. Other have helped in various ways: Paula Falgout shared with me her notes on infertile women of the Bible from a conference she led. Karla Worley and Sandra Davis gave me valuable feedback on several chapters. And Leslie Peacock Caldwell, my editor, friend, and former aerobics buddy, encouraged and advised me along the way.

To the couples who shared their stories, thank you for opening up a part of your life that is, in many cases, painful to remember. Thank you for sharing your crises of faith, your victories, your hopes, your dreams. Your stories represent about sixty lives affected by infertility. In the United States right now, there are more than six million whose stories are not told, not to mention those of past generations who no longer fall into the "Reproductive Age" category. Every story is unique, if we'll just take the time to listen.

Ryan may one day read this book and see his name woven into its stories. He probably won't remember the many times he crawled into my lap and wanted to type on the keyboard as I worked. At least once he banged the keys in some impossible sequence, locking up the keyboard so that I couldn't do anything until Edward came home from work and restored it to normal. When he wasn't trying to take over the keyboard, he would simply sit on my lap and play with the contents of the desk drawer while I tried to look around his curly head to see the computer screen. (I'm not the only writer who had pre-parenthood visions of our children playing quietly on the floor beside our desks as we happily craft novels and other tomes. We learn quickly how pie-in-the-sky that is!) By the end of this book-writing experience, Ryan, who is profoundly deaf, would regularly sign "Mommy works on the computer" when I explained to him that he needed to play with Daddy for the evening. He deserves my thanks for his patient endurance of this prolonged change in his routine.

My prayer is that this book will help you feel camaraderie with other infertility survivors, and that you will feel the freedom to pour out your heart to God during your journey.

# Chapter 1

# Our Story

*In my quiet times this month, I've been drawn to Psalm 139 again und again. I've been impressed to pray this passage for our child, wherever he or she is. "For you created my inmost being; you knit me together in my mother's womb. I praise you because I am fearfully and wonderfully made. . . . My frame was not hidden from you when I was made in the secret place. . . . Your eyes saw my unformed body. All the days ordained for me were written in your book before one of them came to be.* —my journal, August 1997*

Astonishing plots. Complex relationships. Heartbreak and jubilation. Divine intervention. And in many cases, happy endings.

In researching and writing this book, I've heard dozens of true stories from infertile couples. What intrigues me most is the drama inherent to every story. Each infertile couple has a real, live, movie-of-the-week plot unfolding under their own roof. Couples (the protagonists) battle infertility (the antagonist), wrestling with the extremes of human experience—the angst, the euphoria, and all the points in between.

Non-infertile couples? They just get pregnant and have children—how boring is that? (And you're thinking, *Bring on the boredom!*)

When you reach the other side of infertility, you'll have stories of your own. Stories of challenge, disappointment, medical tenacity, weighing options, and eventually resolution. And weaving together the intricacies of your story is our all-knowing, ever-patient Father in heaven.

This is our story—borne of crisis, laced with persistence, and written, we believe, by the hand of God.

## Grand plans

In our pre-infertility days (*"pre"* in the sense that we didn't know we were infertile), my husband Edward and I talked about adopting a child after we'd birthed one or two. Adoption appealed to us. But we never guessed we wouldn't be able to conceive. Not us! Not the seminary graduates, not the couple in ministry.

It was a crisis of identity for me. I had always set goals and been able to reach them. Maybe it was the inner drive of being a firstborn child, but I could look down my life's path and see the string of stars I'd reached. They weren't always lofty goals, but they were *mine*. The dream of becoming a mother seemed easily attainable. Surely I, with my natural instinct for planning, could reach that goal and become a mother when it was realistic, logical, and rational.

But after about five years free of the birth control pill, Edward and I realized that something wasn't working right. I'd read a book about charting my basal body temperature to help me know when I was *not* ovulating. Using that method, we'd avoided pregnancy. I was quite proud of myself for solving that little problem and eliminating the need for pills. When we were ready to get pregnant, I just reversed the procedure: mapping my basal body temperature to know when I *was* ovulating. I began to behave as if no problem was too big for me to figure out using the brain God had given me. (In Texas we call this "gettin' too big for your britches.")

My planning went into hyperdrive. I talked to friends who'd taken maternity leave, and began planning for our short-term disability insurance. I figured out a way to actually increase our income if I stayed home during the maximum 12 weeks. With my accrued sick leave plus the short-term disability, I figured we'd come out ahead. My ingenuity amazed even me.

But after a year of sinking money into insurance premiums, I realized I'd put the proverbial cart before the horse. It would have been nice if I'd prayed about it a little more before I signed up for the extra insurance, but instead I saw it as the logical thing to do and sped forward. We hadn't had even a hint of pregnancy after all those temperature charts. It was now time to go to the next level.

## Let the games begin

In my first consultation with my gynecologist, I'll never forget one of his initial pieces of instruction. He said the first way to try to solve infertility would be to increase our frequency of intercourse, ensuring we would hit ovulation at some point. "Every day for the three weeks you're not on your period," he advised, with the straightest face I'd ever seen. I wanted to laugh in his face. These weren't the giggles of an embarrassed girl, but the you've-gotta-be-kidding chuckles of a stressed woman. Our schedules, if nothing else, would make it impossible. Edward's work routine hopped all over the clock. My job as a magazine editor kept me at my desk until after 7:00 P.M., with galleys brought home to proof in my downtime—whatever that was.

The doctor backpedaled when he saw I wasn't enthralled by the prescription. "Well, at least every other day, then."

The increased frequency didn't do us any good. Diagnostic tests began, and my husband Edward checked out fine. His sperm count in one semen sample could father a medium-sized nation. How's that for a sense of power? My tests were much less conclusive. I'd had symptoms of endometriosis for years, so a laparoscopy was done to remove as much as possible. My doctor ranked the pervasiveness as moderate to severe. The next step was Lupron injections for four months to eliminate whatever remained of the disease. If I was ever going to conceive without hormone therapy, then it would happen in the first few months after going off Lupron, before the endometriosis had time to reemerge.

*I went to the ob/gyn today, presumably to talk about starting Lupron in the near future, but he surprised me by saying we could start today. It was an emotional whammy I wasn't expecting. I've so dreaded these injections and the side effects. I got teary and was pretty honest with Dr. G. about my fears. As he left the room to get the nurse he paused, looked kindly at me, and patted my head, as he would a little sister. It was an unusual moment between doctor and patient—I felt emotionally acknowledged. Maybe it was his out-of-the-ordinary response that was so comforting. The injection itself wasn't too terrible, but I was so worked up at the advent of it, I was an emotional mess the rest of the day.* —my journal

Lupron induces a temporary menopause, complete with hot flashes, night sweats, and moodiness. I don't recommend taking it during the summer months! Save your hot flashes for the winter, when you're trying to stay warm anyway! At first I was a little fascinated by the strange sensations. Each hot flash felt like a small bomb exploding, spreading heat like an internal atomic cloud, making me a little too toasty all over. But the fascination didn't last long—it takes only one or two for you to get the idea. I endured them for four months. I'll never forget that summer, in more ways than one!

*Had a strange encounter on a plane today as I flew to the conference. I sat next to a woman, age 39, from Georgia. We talked about trying to have children. She said an old Native American woman once told her that when you want something very badly, "Just wish!" As she hissed those words, she leaned too close to my seat and was uncomfortably in my face, her eyes wide. She really thought "just wishing" was a viable option. I'd have been pregnant years ago if that was all it took.* —my journal

Conception eluded us still, even after the Lupron. Our insurance company wouldn't cover further infertility treatments, so we were thrilled when some infertile friends at church told us about a study group at a fertility clinic that was tracking the effectiveness of Metrodin. If we could get into the group, the treatments would be free. We pinned all our hopes on being in that study group. But from the beginning, it seemed it wasn't meant to be. The clinic needed my medical records, but the ob/gyn's records office took three months to finally get all my records sent. Finally, I got a call from the fertility clinic's head nurse: The severity of my prior endometriosis barred our inclusion in any of the study groups.

Our hopes and plans deflated like an old balloon. After I hung up the phone, I grabbed some tissues and walked to a coworker's office. My journal tells the rest of the story:

*Thankfully, Rhonda was working late. I asked, "Can I talk to you for a minute?" She was sitting on the floor with page proofs spread around her. She looked up, wide-eyed, and said, "Uh-oh, what's wrong?" I closed the door, sat on the floor, and told her I'd just been*

*rejected for the study group. I immediately broke down. Rhonda has been through all the ups and downs of infertility, so there wasn't anyone better to talk to me at that moment. I'd talk a while, cry a while, and she'd hug me while I cried. She encouraged me to hang on because she knew exactly what I was feeling, but she also knew that somehow God had a child out there for us. She offered to pray with me. I just nodded as I cried, so she put her hands on my head while she prayed the kindest prayer. She prayed that I would know God's peace, which surpasses understanding. She prayed a lot of other things, but that's what I remember most.*  —*my journal*

Rhonda did the best thing she could do: she held me close and let me cry. No grand advice, no pep talks; she simply shared my grief.

Of all days to get bad news, we picked the worst. Edward had just left that morning for his first official business trip. We couldn't be together to commiserate in this setback. Finally, at about 9:00 P.M., we reached each other by phone. He was alone in his hotel room, and I was alone at home. It was a hard evening for us both. Later I realized that my aloneness made God's presence even more evident. I could find comfort nowhere else but in God. An incredible peace began to settle on me. It was just as Rhonda had prayed.

The next day I felt surprisingly content, despite the fact that a major rug had been pulled out. I realized that three months ago we hadn't even known about the study group. The only thing that had changed was that we weren't going to receive free treatment. I wasn't ready to think about what the next step might be. International adoption? Fertility treatments? Domestic adoption?

*We have a good life together. I don't want us to "embrace the empti-ness" that seems to swallow up some infertile couples. "Empty arms" doesn't mean empty hearts. When a couple desperately wants a child, they begin to think that their life is empty without one. They become completely centered on the quest for a child—financially, emotionally, mentally, spiritually. We don't want that feeling to ever control us. We love our life together and want to always be sat-isfied with it, so that if a child comes along, he or she will be an added blessing.*  — *my journal*

The financial burden would fall completely to us from that point on. It didn't take us long to determine that it was time to move to adoption. We had some money in the bank, but we knew it wouldn't last long if we got to the level of in vitro fertilization (IVF) at about ten thousand dollars a cycle. Edward and I are inherently pragmatic. As we reasoned it, we had a sure thing with adoption—eventually we'd be matched with a child, whereas infertility treatments are the technical equivalent of gambling, in our opinion. We determined our money was better invested in adoption.

Frightened by the media's overemphasis on birth parents reclaiming adopted children, we first explored international adoption. It would cost more, but it seemed safer. We began saving money, anticipating we'd need about twenty- to twenty-five thousand dollars. Russia was our first choice; Romania, our second. I found a verse that seemed to confirm our international adoption pursuits: "Do not be afraid, for I am with you; I will bring your children from the east and gather you from the west" (Isaiah 43:5). Russia and Romania were definitely east, and we would come from the west to get there. How providential!

But God was about to intervene in a dramatic way to shift us from international to domestic adoption, an option we thought we'd never consider. And our child would still come from the East.

### Wrong number

Right before Christmas 1996, Edward's mother, Sandra, got the strangest phone call of her life. It was a woman in another state trying to reach an adoption agency. Jill (not her real name), was 29, three months pregnant, and the mother of three children (she had already placed another child through adoption). Sandra explained that this was *not* the number of an adoption agency, and asked what number she was trying to call. The number Jill gave in no way resembled Sandra's number. The only thing they could figure was that the phone call had somehow been rerouted—maybe miraculously? Sandra explained cautiously that she knew of a couple considering adoption that she could put Jill in contact with.

Domestic adoption was *not* what we wanted to pursue; but

what if God wanted to drop this baby into our laps? We couldn't live with ourselves if we didn't explore the possibility. We contacted Vicky Payne, our friend who had started a Christian adoption agency. Vicky took over communicating with Jill, protecting us from the emotional manipulation that some birth parents wage. Jill began pressing Vicky for monthly financial assistance. This was where we saw the true value of an agency interceding for an adoptive couple.

A private investigator located the birth father. Mark (not his real name) believed Jill was prostituting herself on the side, as she often had more money than a waitress could make. Mark also believed that Jill had become pregnant before she moved in with him, and was fingering him as the father in order to reap future child support. He said he would gladly sign parental release documents because he believed it wasn't his child. On the other hand, if it was his child he wouldn't sign. Red flag.

### A change of plans

Almost two months into this tentative relationship, Vicky recommended that the three of us take a trip to visit Jill and begin solidifying the adoption plan. Jill acted excited about our visit.

Once we landed in Jill's state, she changed her tune. We called ahead to let her know we'd arrived, but she began side-stepping the plans, claiming she needed to pick up her son several hours away. Vicky reminded her that this meeting had been planned for several weeks, and Jill acquiesced. We were less than an hour from her home, so we headed quickly in her direction.

We arrived at Jill's mobile home on a quiet street in a small town. No car was in the driveway, no children playing in the sunshine. Jill and her children were gone. Vicky conveyed her concern about these red flags. Although she is a firm believer in open adoption where birth and adopted parents meet and communicate, her evaluation of this situation was that it should be a closed adoption with little interaction between the birth mother and us, if it went through at all.

Vicky decided to track down Mark, who lived in a rougher part of town. She talked with him outside his trailer while we sat in the car (gladly!), and he signed the parental release papers, confirming again that he wasn't the birth father. Then he said something that blew apart our future plans with Jill. He mentioned to Vicky that he had received papers from another agency. He disappeared into the trailer for a few minutes, then brought back a legal-sized envelope: Jill was making an adoption plan with two agencies in two states. She had promised her unborn child to two families!

Our decision was easy: We would not pursue this adoption. Jill was clearly not to be trusted. I had horrible images of two infertile couples showing up at the hospital during Jill's delivery. No, we would back out now. We never even met Jill.

The next day Vicky called Jill to let her know that her commitment to the other agency was out of the bag. Jill invented an excuse, but Vicky announced to her that we were breaking the match. Jill became angry, cursing and shouting so loudly that Edward and I could hear most of what she was yelling into the phone.

Vicky remained calm. Because she directs a Christian adoption agency, she's committed to sharing Christ with birth parents whenever possible. She'd left a Bible after talking with Mark. Now Vicky turned the conversation away from the adoption and toward eternal matters. Jill calmed down, and Vicky was able to present the gospel to Jill over the phone.

Edward and I had prayed God would use the trip to either open the door very widely or close it completely shut. Our prayer had been answered. We left, knowing that this was definitely not the child God intended for us. We could only pray that Jill would place her child with the other agency, for the child's sake.

## A necessary detour

There was some letdown in the weeks to come, but mostly relief. The hardest part was retelling the trip's outcome again and again. Couples who encounter failed fertility treatments know the difficulty of repeating bad news.

Edward's mother was disappointed. She had so hoped God might give us a child as a result of that strange phone call. "It was the first time in my life I truly felt I was part of a miracle," she said. But in a very real way, she was. We look at the failed adoption with no remorse or pain. We see, instead, that it was a necessary piece of our parenting puzzle. We'd been totally focused on international adoption, but God was leading us to switch directions. The episode with Jill spurred us to connect with Vicky and fill out our adoption paperwork. God needed us to be in a position to accept what He was going to give us just one year later, almost to the day. With all our paperwork completed at Vicky's agency, we asked her to keep showing our biographical profile to birth mothers.

### Moving forward, moving west

Edward's career moved us from Alabama to Texas that summer, and we were consumed with selling our house, packing, moving, and looking for a new home in a new city. All this activity was a godsend to keep our minds off infertility for about six months. In August 1997, in the midst of transition between the two states, God brought my attention to Psalm 139. I felt that somewhere a child existed, born or unborn, and that child was meant to be ours.

In September 1997, out of the blue, Edward's Aunt Dianne called to say she knew of a pregnant teenager living with a family at her church. The 17-year-old girl was thinking about adoption, so interested couples were showering her with biographical profile sheets to consider. If we were interested, ours could be added to the pile.

"But don't get your hopes up," Dianne warned. We sent our one-page profile, in which we described ourselves, our interests, our faith, and our dreams for being parents. We also mentioned how much we like Winnie the Pooh. When I was 17, I regarded persons in their mid-30s as knocking on the door of middle age. I included a picture of us in matching Mickey Mouse shirts, hoping it would emphasize our youthfulness! It seemed pretty silly, but that picture would play a part in our future.

We heard nothing for months. We closed on our Texas home and began extensive remodeling. For two months I caulked, cleaned, and painted. The time alone gave me hundreds of hours to think about where our lives were going. Many times I found myself praying for that young mother-to-be who was trying to decide about adoption. We only knew she was due in late January, nothing else. I had no idea what her situation was, whether or not she was a Christian, nothing. I prayed for her salvation and for her child to one day come to know Christ. I prayed that whomever she chose would give the child a godly home. If we couldn't raise her child, at least I could pray for those who would.

November came, and it was time to get all the furniture out of storage and finally move into our completed home. We had convinced ourselves that the girl had probably chosen another couple from her stack of profiles. If only we could know for sure, though, we could emotionally close that book and move forward. We reminded ourselves, however, that we don't always have the privilege of knowing how things resolve, and that we might never know how this one ended. But it was hard to put it out of our minds, try as we might.

## Caught between joy and devastation

As the Christmas season rolled in, I relished the chance to dote on my two-year-old nephew, Alexander, who lived in the same town. Being able to "borrow" someone else's child once in while helps you fulfill some of your parental longings. We took Alexander to see Christmas decorations at an amusement park, where we ate huge gingerbread cookies. And Edward and I hung up our stockings for our ninth Christmas together—trying not to dwell on having another year with no child's stocking beside our own.

Alexander became a big brother in January. What makes little Timothy's birth date so significant to our story is the emotional polarities we experienced the day he was born. I planned to see him and his parents at the hospital that afternoon, and knew I would need to bolster my emotional reserves for the afternoon visit: any time I was around babies it was an emotional whammy.

The day grew even more complicated just a few hours before my trip to the hospital. I learned from Edward's mother that the pregnant teen had actually liked our profile most of all. She called us "those Disney people," and was drawn to the photo of our Mickey shirts and our fondness for Pooh. Though due in January, she'd had a C-section in early November due to preeclampsia. She had almost died, and the baby had to be taken quickly. Her tiny son was born at 26 weeks weighing only 1 pound, 6.2 ounces, 11½ inches long. He was still in the neonatal intensive care unit (NICU) on oxygen and monitors, fighting for his life. The mother had decided to keep him; though if she had placed for adoption *she would have chosen us.*

*She would have chosen us.* It echoed in our minds, stabbing us deeper each time. We were devastated.

Sitting in the hospital room that mid-January afternoon, I held my brand-new nephew and thanked God for his little life. But my emotions were a jumbled mess. I had promised myself I wouldn't mention our new disappointment to my brother and sister-in-law. It was a big day for them. So I just held Timothy and rocked him gently. But I couldn't keep from wondering why God was letting life run over us like this.

**New choices**

Just two weeks later, Edward and I sat staring at the menu of our favorite restaurant. Would we order the same old thing or try something new? Before the evening was over, it was clear that the routines in our life would never be the same again.

While waiting for dinner to arrive, Edward's pager went off. It was a message from Dianne: "Call me when you both can talk." We got to-go boxes and headed home. Dianne definitely had news: The young mother was vacillating in her decision about keeping the baby. Were we still interested?

Absolutely! The baby boy was still in the NICU, and would be for several more weeks. The birth mom was weighing her decision but leaning toward adoption. Her concern was if anyone would be willing to take a baby with so many potential problems. For some reason that I cannot attribute to our logical natures, we were drawn to this fragile child. God must have been weaving this little one into our hearts before we even met him. We determined to walk through this door and just see what would happen.

From the outset, we knew this baby would be high maintenance. Having been born so early, he was naturally at risk for developmental delays, cerebral palsy, hearing/eyesight disorders, physical/motor delays, and more. We approached the decision with prayer and education. We began learning everything we could about the long-term effects of prematurity. We searched the Internet, chatted online with parents of preemies, and called NICU nurses for advice.

The more we learned, the more we were amazed that this child was even alive. The threshold for survivability at that time was 26 weeks (with a 23-week gestational age). There was no good reason why the child hadn't died, especially since some whopping infections had attacked his immunity-deprived system.

The birth mom vacillated in her decision for several weeks, for which I can't blame her. She had bonded emotionally with her child in the months since his birth. She went to see him every single day at the hospital. She loved him. She wanted to keep him. But she was seriously considering whether or not a teenaged girl who hadn't even graduated from high school could effectively provide for the multitude of needs this child would have.

February rolled along, and several times she decided to keep him. Then she would be at the other end of the spectrum. All this time the baby was in the hospital. On February 20 she brought him home from the hospital to live in her room—oxygen tanks, apnea monitors, and all.

On March 1 we received a phone call that would seal our fate. The birth mom had determined, after having the baby home and caring for him herself, that there was no way she could give him what he needed while trying to prepare herself for a productive future as a single, working mom. It was just too much to handle. As much as she loved him and wanted to keep him, she chose his needs above her desires. She wanted us to come get her baby as soon as possible.

Just a few days later I was on a plane with Vicky, headed to meet this brave teenager who would entrust us with the most precious possession of her young life. Almost immediately after we arrived she asked me timidly, "Do you want to hold the baby?" "Oh, can I?" I asked incredulously. At four months, he was still only five pounds, sixteen inches long. She carefully laid in my arms the little boy we would name Ryan, keeping the birth name she had given him, Benjamin, as a middle name.

Over the next few days we were in an intense learning

curve, becoming familiar with the apnea monitor, pulse oximeter, and oxygen tank—not to mention the normal steps of feeding and caring for a fragile infant. When the young woman officially relinquished her parental rights, she gave us a photo album of the baby's first few months, along with the letter she had written for his benefit in the years to come:

*You were home about a week when I decided that I was going to place you up for adoption. I was scared that I wouldn't always be able to supply you with all of the medical stuff that you needed. The couple your father and I chose for you were the only couple we had looked at the whole time. They are a very down-to-earth couple and I trust them. I feel they can provide you with what your father and I cannot. You deserve the world. Your father and I love you a lot and we will never forget you, son. Always remember that. We didn't place you for adoption because we don't love you. We did it because we do.*

## Life with Ryan

That's our happy ending, or actually our happy beginning. But then an unbelievable sequel began unfolding just four months after we had Ryan at home. Unbeknownst to Ryan's birth mother, the neonatologist, or any of the half-dozen specialists who had cared for him, there were medical issues in his little body that we believe God was shielding from discovery until after he was placed with us. If we had known about these issues at the time of placement, we might have been too practical to proceed. We might have assumed that God had another couple, a medically savvy one, who would come out of nowhere. God knew us well: We wouldn't trust ourselves to take on such a challenge. But God trusted us.

In June, a neurologist ordered a CAT scan—a routine test for preemies who are at risk for underdeveloped brains. No one expected to find calcium deposits in that little head. He'd had several cranial sonograms in NICU, but that level of testing doesn't reveal calcium deposits. Calcium deposits can cause a long list of developmental problems, and we cried many tears as our understanding of Ryan's future became cloudy. I sat in his room many nights rocking him to sleep with silent tears inching down my face, begging God to let his neural pathways form over and around those deposits.

In August, a routine set of X-rays revealed another hidden anomaly: unusually shaped vertebrae, a condition unnoticed even though Ryan had had dozens of chest X-rays in the NICU. A half-dozen orthopedic specialists around the country arrived at the diagnosis of dyssegmental dysplasia. This autosomal recessive trait is a dwarfism syndrome. In every documented case (only about 40 in 40 years), it has been fatal before age three.

Suddenly, the calcium deposits didn't seem so bad after all. Edward and I were told that Ryan was already an exception to the rule—he was fairly healthy, whereas other victims have lung complications that eventually lead to their demise. "We'll just have to wait and let Ryan show us what he is going to do," the doctors said.

We were just coming to terms with that diagnosis when a hearing test revealed that Ryan was profoundly deaf, probably caused by some of the meds he had been given in NICU. "The deafness will affect him far more than the dwarfism," the orthopedist told us. We came to realize that our own birth child could have just as many medical problems since no one knows what syndromes lie hidden in the chromosomes (at least not yet).

## No mistakes, no regrets
Those were the darkest days of our lives as new parents. After more than nine years of infertility, we were aghast that God would ask us to deal with this too. Didn't we deserve a normal parenthood after all that suffering?

As we began living with all these diagnoses we gained new friends in Ryan's pulmonologist, neurologist, audiologist, geneticist, orthopedist, otolaryngologist, three therapists (physical, occupational, and speech), plus his pediatrician. Our lives became far more complicated (medically) than we'd imagined possible. But in a dozen other ways, we were enjoying Ryan's infancy immensely.

Never once, even in the midst of the horrible diagnoses, did we have the tiniest regret that we'd adopted Ryan. We'd do it again in a flash. The circumstances that led us to Ryan were divine, and we were sure that this was no mistake.

Infertility

## God's grace

The storm clouds of that first year have lifted, and we are humbled by the grace God has poured out on Ryan. Allow me to use the word *miracle* here. We believe it's a miracle that some of those earlier diagnoses are no longer at the forefront. Our little boy shows no noticeable complications from the calcium deposits. He is developmentally on track, and even began identifying letters of the alphabet before he was three. His dwarfism syndrome is the biggest mystery of all: he shows no external evidence of it. His lungs and skeleton are growing perfectly in tandem, and though he's at the bottom of the growth chart for his age, he's growing at the same rate as other kids.

The deafness occupies our attention now, just as the orthopedist predicted. We're learning sign language, and Ryan takes to it like a fish to water. We've been blessed with extended family members who constantly support and encourage us. They are learning sign language so they can talk to Ryan without going through us as interpreters.

When Ryan meets people, he looks to us and asks their name in sign language. Then he wants to know where they keep their vacuum cleaner! He's fascinated by machines. When someone comes to visit, he thinks it's his inalienable right to sit in their car and pretend to drive, curiously turning every knob and pressing all the buttons. He is delightfully normal in so many ways.

Edward and I look at Ryan and marvel. It's a miracle he's in our lives; it's a miracle he's alive; and it's a miracle he's thriving so well.

*I can look back and see God's hand in our journey. His providential guidance is evident in countless ways when we stop and consider all He has done to allow Ryan to be placed in our home.*  —Edward

In spite of our infertility, we have been blessed indeed.

# Chapter 2

# A Woman's Perspective on Infertility

*During our infertility journey, I wondered, "What have I done that would make God not give me a baby? Am I somehow unfit, and He's protecting an innocent life from me? Is there some sin I haven't confessed? Why can everyone else have a baby whenever they want? What about all those girls having babies they can't care for, or those having abortions?" I never dreamed of being a teacher or doctor or lawyer or anything but a mom. I couldn't reconcile my dreams of motherhood with the reality I was living.* —Angela

You're not alone. Let it sink in. *You are not alone.* Almost every woman I've talked to has felt alone at some point in her infertility struggle. Even if you know other women who have struggled, you may feel that you're the only person who has faced this variation of infertility. And, well, that's a little bit true. Your infertility is unlike my infertility, and my infertility is unlike Angela's. Infertility cuts us off from each other, but mostly it cuts us off from the self we used to know and the dreams we grew up with.

But we can find strength in knowing about the journeys of other women who walk in the "Valley of Infertility." You'll find that you're not alone in the emotional battle that goes hand in hand with the physical one.

If you're a man involved in this infertility battle, think of this chapter as your wife's way of saying, "Here's what I can't always put into words." The end of this chapter gives some ideas for how a husband can listen and respond to his wife.

## A woman's dreams

(or why infertility gets us down in the first place)

In today's society, where women have almost limitless opportunities for education and career, do women still long for that age-old dream of being a happy wife and mom? You better believe it! Today's woman wants it all—an education, a career, marriage, and motherhood.

The young women who struggle with infertility in our culture have grown up with something other than the Ozzie and Harriet model for a home life. We know women don't always get married right after high school, pop out a handful of babies, and settle into the roles of homemaker, room mother, and carpooler. Women have many additional options to choose from—and our career roles aren't limited to teacher, nurse, or secretary anymore. We can point to female astronauts who have children, to senators and entrepreneurs who have both family and career. We know female lawyers who've started a family, then chosen to stay home full time. We know of marriages where both partners work in medicine. We see women serving in ministry, in the military, in public office—women in every imaginable field.

And yet for most women, alongside the dream to spend a little time or a long time in a rewarding career, there's the enduring desire to be a mother. The fires that liberated women's educational and employment options didn't singe our desire to hold our babies close to our hearts and whisper lullabies in their ears until they fall asleep. The desire to be a mom still runs strong and deep.

*I grew up with a mental schedule of how my life would progress: Get an education, work for a while, and then stay home with children. Unconsciously, part of my dream was the expectation that I'd be in control of where, when, and how I became a mother.*

*—my journal*

When that dream eludes our grasp, when we find that we're infertile, we're more than a little frustrated and disappointed: We're downright shocked! We've been raised to believe we can set goals and reach them. We can get an education or job training and achieve a career goal. We can control whom we marry. We can control our destiny by our commitment to hard work and our dedication to the task.

*How could this happen to me? I've played by the rules. I've gotten my education. I've worked and matured. I'm ready now for a family. We're ready to be parents. Why is this being denied us?*

*—my journal*

Infertility, however, doesn't play by the same rulebook. Infertility doesn't even *have* a rulebook. Infertility is, for most of us, the most formidable opponent we've ever encountered. It doesn't respond to logic, rational planning, strategic thinking, or investigative research. Two women can have similar infertility problems and be treated with identical protocols. One will get pregnant and the other won't. Infertility is a tough egg to crack (pardon the pun).

### So we're a little naive

American women are especially likely to think pregnancy and family planning will come together easily and within a predictable time frame. Born in the mid- to latter part of the twentieth century, we rarely consider the family model that existed for generations—when women bore numerous children (no birth control existed other than abstinence) and women frequently lost one or more children, due to childhood diseases and less sophisticated medical care.

Yet that model isn't so far removed from us. Our grandparents were the first generation to birth children who almost assuredly lived to adulthood, due to improved health care available in the early and mid–20th century. But go back one more generation, when the mothers of pre-20th-century America were bearing children sometimes annually and losing several along the way to birth complications or childhood illnesses. No one assumed they were exempt from the heartache of losing children. It was a part of life. They weren't naive enough to think that tragedy would bypass them.

As women born in post-World War II America, we assume the complete opposite: We think we're in charge of our family planning just as much as every other aspect of our lives. When the truth hits us, our lack of control over our destiny rocks our world.

*We believed that in spite of my age of 38 and Joe's age of 40, we would have little trouble getting pregnant. Looking back on it, I can't imagine why we felt this way. Perhaps it was a way of denying the cold, biological fact that we were growing older and our chances for conceiving and bearing children had slipped away.*     —*Jan*

## What we feel

Disappointment, frustration, confusion, anger, disbelief, fear—the darkest gamut of human emotions wash over a woman.

*I always assumed I'd be able to get pregnant at the time of my choosing. I was in shock when it didn't happen. I felt inadequate and frustrated. I withdrew emotionally and socially. And I mourned.*
     —*Paula*

*My mother started menopause at 31. I knew the odds were 50 percent that I would start menopause in my thirties. Since I was twenty-seven at the time, I felt an urgency to get pregnant so we would have time to have two children.*     —*Christy*

*I always thought that the ability to bear children is what makes a woman wholly unique—and I couldn't even do that.*     —*Linda*

Early on, Ann and Wallace weren't too concerned that they weren't getting pregnant. "But when the testing started and we flunked every test, it got very *real* very *fast*, and we were immediately faced with the words, 'There's a good chance you will not have children.'"

Those words shatter the fragile dreams a woman has for motherhood. Most of us can remember the day we heard words like that. For some women, though, it's a slow dawning of a grim reality. A doctor may not come right out and brand you as infertile; but as the months and the tests pass and the results don't go as hoped, you begin to realize that you share the unpleasant label of infertility with a group of people who never thought they'd be infertile, either.

*Like the rest of the world, we thought that when it was time to start a family we would just get pregnant and have children. We both*

*tried to be patient, knowing that God really did have our best inter-
ests in His heart. But there were still many tears, many sleepless
nights, and about a million people who had "suggestions" for us.
We were scared. We wondered if our dreams of being parents would
never come true.* —Dinah

Who knows if it's a genetic thing, but women have a natural tendency to compare themselves to each other. We all do
it. And infertility makes it all the worse because now we're
comparing ourselves to every woman who is currently pregnant or who has ever been pregnant, which means we have
ample opportunity to feel like we're less than normal.

*We start competing with other women when the race to get engaged
begins. At least, it did in my generation in the mid-1970s. When
you got engaged, you stepped into another "category" that separated
you from the rest of the pack. Then, marriage put you into a different group, one that's racing to start having children. How you carried off your pregnancy and childbirth was competition, too.
Infertility has its own competitiveness. There's all this "sisterhood"
among women who are going through the same tests and procedures. But when one gets pregnant, she "graduates." And though
you're happy for her, you are left behind.* —Karla

### That monthly crushing blow

Infertility is frequently called an emotional roller coaster.
Every month, a woman has another chance to soar with joy or
plummet to the depths of despair.

*You think every month will be the month. You live in a cycle of
anticipation and hope, followed by crushing disappointment.*
—Angela

I grew up knowing that my Aunt Ellen and Uncle Paul had
two adopted children. Not that it mattered to me that they
were adopted, but it was just a fact comfortably acknowledged in our family. But it wasn't until I was writing this
book that it dawned on me: Aunt Ellen and Uncle Paul had
faced infertility, too. When I asked Aunt Ellen about it, she
said her heart would break every month:

*When I would cry at the time of my menses, Paul would always hold me and say, "Honey, I married you because I love you. If we have children, that's great, but I'd rather have you than anyone." Sometimes it would console me and sometimes not. I wanted to be content with Paul, but I also wanted a child.*

When our quest for children becomes public knowledge, well-meaning friends and family show they care by asking for regular updates. This has its pluses and minuses.

*We were everybody's project. Every month, they asked, "So . . . are you?" Dennis hated that part of it. I didn't want to be part of a "club" for women with infertility. I didn't want to compare test results and hear details of their laparoscopies. I've seen women tell perfect strangers all the gory details of their pregnancies and give them advice. Infertile women are subjected to the same thing.*

—*Karla*

## Unprepared for battle

When two people marry and neither has been married before, you can ask them what they know about marriage, and they'll tell you. But none of it comes from personal experience, only observation. Likewise, when a woman learns she's infertile, she has no personal experience to benefit her. But as infertility has come to the surface of public awareness, more women know of others who've walked this road before. Not too long ago, almost no one admitted to infertility.

*Information was scarce and usually contradictory when we began battling infertility in the 1980s. No one we knew could relate to what we were experiencing. It was a very lonely time. (Angela)*

Consider, too, that the women who face infertility for the first time are young—anywhere from the early twenties and up. They don't have the life experience to handle crises with emotional balance, as an older woman might. Infertility strikes women who are least equipped to handle it emotionally. Once women hit their mid-thirties, they expect to experience decreased fertility in some way, through most women feel they are still in control of their reproductive potential.

*In my early thirties, I expected it might take us a year or two to get pregnant on our own, and that we'd need to pay attention to when I was most likely ovulating; but surely it could happen without intervention. I mean, we're both healthy, active adults. Now, at thirty-six, I am still childless without so much as a hint of a conception to my name. I feel like my pursuit of motherhood has hit a brick wall.*

*—my journal*

One of the best ways for a woman to survive infertility's battles is to find one or two other women who have experienced infertility.

*We had some very close friends who had gone through infertility. It was an amazing comfort to have them to lean on and bounce things off of. They unselfishly shared their stories with us, and for this we will be ever grateful.* *—Dinah*

Because of the prevalence of infertility today, it's a lot easier to find someone else who knows of its struggles. Most people cluster in informal groups for mutual encouragement—lunch together, a phone call, girls' night out—but organized support groups exist around the country. The most well known is RESOLVE (see "Resources" at the end of this book). Or look on the Internet for virtual communities of fellow strugglers. By searching under "Infertility," I found a number of Web sites established by women who had experienced all levels of treatment and knew firsthand about the pain. Some of the sites offer message boards, through which you can communicate with other women.

### What women think of their bodies

We come to adulthood expecting our bodies to do what we want, when we want; but when it doesn't work that way, we can feel shortchanged, tricked, betrayed by the very body we inhabit.

*Betrayed was exactly how I felt. I assumed because I had always been healthy and strong and came from a big family, I would have no trouble conceiving and carrying to term. My first son was conceived with no trouble, but he died while trying to be born from my body, and that made it all the worse. I felt responsible for his death, and on some levels I will always feel that way.*                                    —*Cathy*

Youthful women are accustomed to pushing their bodies to the limit and getting the maximum benefit and accomplishments—exercise, work responsibilities, college courses, church responsibilities, and more. We (that is, our minds) used to be in control of determining our future, but now the tables have turned. Some faulty aspect of our bodies is in control of our future and whether or not we'll be able to birth a child. We can't just push ourselves a little longer and harder, as we might do with an exercise routine. We can't stay up later and work longer hours to find the answer. Our bodies have created a silent, invisible, elusive lock that keeps us from getting pregnant, and we search for the right key to match. We are helpless to fix the problem in our own power, and that's hard to swallow.

*Early in our infertility work-up, it was determined that the problem was with me, even though no one knew what the problem was. I remember wishing so badly that I could know what was going wrong inside my body so that it could be corrected and we could have a child.*                                    —*Linda*

*I felt like I was doing everything wrong. Maybe I wasn't taking good care of myself. Maybe I should lose more weight. Maybe I'm the one who needs to just relax, like everyone says, and it will happen. I beat myself up pretty badly at times.*                                    —*Dinah*

*I thought because I'd had so many miscarriages and an operation to remove cysts from my ovaries, that my body was telling me that I was an unfit mother. It was a very painful time in my life. Even when I conceived again, I didn't tell our family for several months, as I was so afraid of miscarrying and being a failure once again.*
                                    —*Debbie*

*I felt like Pat, the genderless character on Saturday Night Live. I couldn't do what a woman should be able to do. I had feelings of inadequacy. I felt I was not as good as women who could reproduce.*
                                    —*Ann*

Another big question is "Why me?" Christian women especially may feel they've abided by the rules God sets forth in His Word for moral behavior in premarital relationships, and therefore should be able to bear children as a guaranteed benefit of such obedience.

*I always thought infertility happened to other people, not people like us. What did I do to deserve this? I always did as I was told. I never got into any major trouble, so why was God punishing me? I looked at all the teenagers with children, homeless people who kept having children, abusive people who had unwanted children. We were very capable of being parents and we were being denied this privilege.*

—Celeste

## And then we beat ourselves up

When the infertility problem lies with the woman's reproductive system, she often feels she's depriving her husband of a family. And though her husband may be quick to refute her opinion, she still harbors guilt. Some women, in fits of self-deprecating anger, even encourage their husbands to find a new wife who can give them children. "I felt like I was cheating my husband out of a family," Linda says. She battled feelings of unfairness and guilt. Beth knew how much Joel longed to be a father, "and that added to the stress I felt." Feelings of inadequacy hit hard.

*I felt like I wasn't worthy as a woman and a wife. Women are supposed to have children. We are the ones who bring life. My body was not succeeding, so I considered myself a failure.* —Christy

*We've been able to birth one child, but we're still dealing with infertility. I feel extremely guilty because the problem lies with me. Mike is perfectly healthy and normal. I sometimes feel that if Mike had married someone else, he would have had all the children he wanted; but because of me, we will only have one child. Mike is so wonderful, though. He says all the time that, no matter what, he didn't want to marry anyone else; and if Briley is the only child we have, we are truly blessed to have him, and he is completely happy with that.* —Celeste

Women have a tendency to find their value in the roles they assume. Where men often find value in the work they do, their wives find value in who they see themselves to be. Though we may have an identity in the workplace, many of us still grow up feeling an unconscious pull to be a wife and mom. Women who never marry and never become mothers may struggle with finding self-worth. The same is true for women who, though married, are thwarted in their childbearing efforts.

A woman's self-worth and self-image spiral downward as a result of infertility. Test after test increases the pace of the plummet. Failed cycles and miscarriages multiply the miserable opinion we have of ourselves.

**Immerse yourself in God's love**
Yet God never once said that He places value on what we do, who we are, what roles we manage to secure, or the number of children we produce. His value system bestows on us a worth above any of those: "I have loved you with an everlasting love" (Jeremiah 31:3). God loves us because we are His precious children.

I would often read Psalm 139, especially verses 13 through 16, and pray for the child that God would bring to us one day. Then my friend Paula shared with me an insight I had missed:

*I became very convicted when I read about being "fearfully and wonderfully made." I'd had such tunnel vision that all I could think about was my inability to produce good eggs and get pregnant. I apologized to God in a big way and started thanking God for the countless parts of my body that worked well, but that I had overlooked.* —Paula

Call on the Word of God to lift you up during this time of self-devaluation. You are precious in God's sight just as you are. Let His love permeate your brokenness as you read these verses.

*"The Lord is close to the brokenhearted and saves those who are crushed in spirit."* —*Psalm 34:18*

*"He heals the brokenhearted and binds up their wounds."*
*—Psalm 147:3*

*"This is how God showed his love among us: He sent his one and only Son into the world that we might live through him. This is love: not that we loved God, but that he loved us and sent his Son as an atoning sacrifice for our sins."* *—1 John 4:9–10*

*"And so we know and rely on the love God has for us. God is love. Whoever lives in love lives in God, and God in him. In this way, love is made complete among us so that we will have confidence on the day of judgment, because in this world we are like him. There is no fear in love. But perfect love drives out fear, because fear has to do with punishment. The one who fears is not made perfect in love. We love because he first loved us."* *—1 John 4:16–19*

*"May our Lord Jesus Christ himself and God our Father, who loved us and by his grace gave us eternal encouragement and good hope, encourage your hearts and strengthen you in every good deed and word."* *—2 Thessalonians 2:16–17*

### Tips for husbands who love their wives
Husbands often say they feel helpless to know how to help their wives during the infertility struggle.

Here are some suggestions:

**1. Resist the approach: "Honey, let's tackle this problem and solve it quickly."** This mentality doesn't work with infertility. Infertility requires being a detective in a pitch-dark warehouse trying to find a hidden light switch with one short match. Most women I've talked with say their husbands wanted to tackle the infertility problem quickly and get it fixed. Your wife needs you to recognize and respect the seriousness of the problem. A hurry-up attitude seems to belittle the severity of it.
*We were both frustrated, but Ben was ready to move much quicker than I was. I went through an anger and frustration stage toward Ben. He was pushing so hard for fertility treatments, and I resented the pushing. I would have been happy to adopt right then.* *—Sherri*

*2. Anticipate the things that will remind her of childlessness.*
When you're both out in public, be alert for pregnant women,
parents with little children, baby stores in the mall, or children's playgrounds. Remember that every time she sees them,
it stabs her heart. Give her hand an extra squeeze. Make eye
contact, even if you don't say a thing. She needs to know that
you understand how seeing these reminders hurts deeply,
and she needs to know that it hurts you, too. Let her know
you understand what's going through her mind. (See chapter
5: "Why Do They Have Children and We Don't?")

*3. Hug her and hold her, especially when she cries.* Your
embrace does a world of good, even though it won't stop her
crying. A simple phrase like "I'm sorry we're going through
this" can help her sense the shared aspect of the infertility
burden. Another good one is "I'll always love you no matter
what." Let her cry—don't tell her when it's time to stop. She'll
know when she's finished. Processing grief can't be a scheduled activity. The grief of infertility is something you both
must learn to live with while you try to solve the problem.

*4. Let your wife vent her emotions, even though may feel
helpless to make it better.* She's got to vent somewhere; and
if you make it uncomfortable for her to have an outlet with
you, she'll scrunch it all up internally. And if she keeps it all
inside, you can bet it'll come forth some other time like an
erupting volcano, like when you leave yesterday's socks on
the floor. Even if she vents to friends, it's not the same as talking with you, her soul mate. Listen with your ears and your
eyes (eye contact is a biggie for women), not while you do the
bills, watch the news, glance through a sports magazine, or
spend time on the computer. This is not the time to multitask.
Getting the wrong response from you can be more painful
than not getting any response. If the two of you don't have a
track record for effective communication, she may think she'll
risk less pain by not sharing with you the innermost emotions
of her heart. But she needs to share.

As you listen, don't tell her how she should feel ("Don't let
it get you down so much"). Don't try to talk her out of hurting ("Come on, it's not the end of the world"). Don't try to

solve the problem for her, unless she's asking you directly for answers. Most of the time, she just needs you to listen and to assure her that you're 100 percent with her in this.

5. *Channel your energies usefully.* To be fair to you men, we women need some of your action-oriented response in the midst of tragedy, even though we need it in small, carefully measured doses. If you want to confront your challenger (infertility) with a reservoir of ammunition (I mean, information), get on the Internet and find resources and Web sites that will increase your understanding of the specific infertility problems you're facing. Go to the library or the bookstore. You may need to acquire the information to feel like you're doing something, but she may not have that same need. Ask her if she'd like to read what you've printed out, what books you found, what magazine article you ran across. Maybe she'd rather you simply summarize it for her at first. Make it available to her and she'll read it when she's emotionally ready.

6. *Being there means being there, literally.* Women are subjected to a dizzying array of tests, procedures, injections, ultrasounds, and more—usually alone. Go with her to appointments whenever you can. The moral support is priceless.

*As much as possible, attend appointments as a couple. I realize this may not always be realistic, but the companionship and comfort were a big help. Having a second set of ears present to question the doctor and hear his explanations was beneficial, too.* —Paula

While your infertility journey is unique to you, we all stumble over some of the same pitfalls along the way. Nothing can completely take away your pain and frustration. But remember you are not alone, other women are feeling many of the same things, and most important, you are valued and unconditionally loved by your Father.

*Rhonda and Wayne*

# Finding peace, finally

When Rhonda opened the door to greet her date in spring 1974, she knew there must be some mistake. She was looking at Wayne, but wasn't she supposed to go out with Richard? Both men were at her church, but she'd never talked with either in person. When Wayne called and asked her out, she thought it was Richard she was agreeing to go out with. "I had on shoes with a three-inch heel," Rhonda said. "Wayne is five-foot-five, and I was towering over him. I spent the entire evening with my shoulders slumped and my knees bent forward!"

But this comic beginning didn't sabotage their relationship. "By the time the evening was over, we discovered we had so much in common." Nine months later they were married. They wanted "a house full of children"—six would have been perfect. And fourteen months after their wedding, Rhonda was pregnant.

"I nearly went into cardiac arrest fighting the traffic so I could get home to tell Wayne our good news." Wayne was a music minister. The next Sunday, he announced from the pulpit that Rhonda (the pianist) was not alone at the piano, that they were expecting their first child. "I'm sure our expressions were like Gomer Pyle's 'gaaw-lee!' "

Sadly, an emergency trip to the hospital one day revealed a tubal pregnancy. "One day I was going to be a mommy, and the next day it was all over," Rhonda remembers. "The pain, both physically and emotionally, was beyond words."

The tubal pregnancy complicated matters further. Her affected fallopian tube had to be removed. Months later, she was pregnant again, but the bleeding began immediately. "On Wayne's twenty-eighth birthday I was in the emergency room having a D&C." She had miscarried. "This time we really felt slapped in the face. We were hurt, devastated, and unsure of our faith. We were really confused about why God was allowing this to happen."

Procedures, tests, and infertility drugs netted no results. "The drugs were making me crazy, as if I weren't already; and every month if I was a moment late with my period, I'd rush out for a pregnancy test. I was driving myself insane—and Wayne too. Then when I'd take the pregnancy test, I'd die a little inside, knowing another month had come and gone and I was still not pregnant."

Rhonda and Wayne's friendship had always been their strength, but Rhonda began to think that Wayne probably wished he had married someone else who could give him children. "I told him he should leave me and go find someone else. Then I would have times that I wouldn't talk at all, or times when I felt so badly about myself that I'd say things to hurt the people who loved me most, just so they would hurt, too."

They moved to another state to pursue seminary training, and at their new location Rhonda found a gynecologist who was convinced he could help her. It would require surgery to reconstruct all her reproductive organs, medications, and recuperation time. "Whatever he said, I heard it as I would be pregnant. So I was ready." But it didn't happen.

"I thought seminary students should really have their act together and have a clear picture of God. In my pain, my act was not together and my picture of God was about as clear as mud. The struggle took over my life. Getting pregnant was all I could think of and all I could talk about."

A turning point came when her friend Jody asked if they had considered adoption. "It was like a light bulb went on in my head." The next morning, Rhonda called an agency, and two years later Wayne and Rhonda held seven-day-old Matthew in their arms.

Fast-forward.

More than a decade later, at age forty-one, Rhonda was thrilled to learn she was pregnant again. "We'd take pregnancy at any age," she said. But a heartbeat was never heard, even in the third month. "This loss really hit me hardest. I went to bed and thought about staying there forever."

But one afternoon, eleven-year-old Matthew kneeled beside her bed with a freshly picked wildflower in his hand. "He held it out to me and said, 'Here, Mom, I picked this for you. Don't feel bad. You still have me.' Well, that did it! I got up from my bed, picked myself up, and started all over again."

But the allure of pregnancy called to her again. "The doctors said I only had a 10 percent chance of ever getting pregnant. But, hey, it was 10 percent!" This time she took the strongest fertility drugs and endured shots, tests, exams, and more. "The expenses were draining us, but I didn't care. We maxed-out all the credit cards and had more debt than anyone can imagine. But I would have gone from bank to bank for loans if it took it." Six months and nothing.

"Finally, one morning after sitting in the waiting room, I decided I just couldn't do this anymore. I had the usual ultrasound, then walked to my car, got inside, and cried my eyes out. In that parking lot, I surrendered this pregnancy thing once and for all. And for the first time in my life, I felt a peace—a real peace about my life and who I was. God had given me so much, and now it was time for me to focus on that."

Rhonda drove home in tears—happy tears. She put behind her the three failed pregnancies, and began to look forward. "We had lots of bills to pay back, and it took a long time, but our new life together as a family was beginning. And together, we could make it."

# Chapter 3

# A Man's Perspective on Infertility

**by Edward Dake**

*I think men are just as excited to start families as women are, but they aren't as emotional in the process. In the same manner, men simply aren't as emotional in their coping as they are rational. Therefore, when the situation was becoming clear that we did indeed have an infertility issue, my reaction was more, "What can I do to support Angela?" The actual emotions were a sense of failure, inadequacy, and being somewhat less than a man. However, that rational side of being a man took over and simply steered my focus toward solving the problem.*

*—Jim*

Five years. Our goal was to be married five years and then start a family. We succeeded in waiting a little more than five years, then ended up waiting five more before the adoption of our son, Ryan.

Those first five years were filled with normal, married couple occurrences. Then came the time when both Cindy and I felt we were ready to start a family. That isn't to say that I leapt into this with abandon. I moved glacially into being ready to become a father. Since my preparation and my thinking were slow to come around, once I did reach the *feeling* that it was okay to start a family, I expected it to happen quickly.

When our attempts fell short of producing even a false hope of pregnancy, the roller-coaster ride began. The emotional experience that ensued was a lot like a roller-coaster ride I remember that occurred entirely inside a large building and completely in the dark. There were curves I didn't see coming. There were lurching, dramatic drop-offs that took me by surprise. There were slow, agonizing climbs that built anticipation of a thrill at the other side, but flattened out to disappointment; but unlike the theme park ride, there wasn't the over-too-soon ending to the emotions that accompanied our infertility journey.

I felt alienated from friends, from God, from family that I felt couldn't understand our trials. I felt I stood alone in the howling winds of this storm and, at any moment, I knew those winds might rip me off the face of this planet.

What men experience during infertility is almost always considered secondary to anything that women encounter. And, as Jim says, men generally assume the role of supporting and encouraging their wives, which is certainly needed. But this chapter will explore much more than that. Men who lock horns with infertility have battles of their own—battles that demand more from them than society gives them credit for enduring. They deal with true pain when faced with the fact that they may not be a father. And they may deal with specific issues, such as feeling loss, sadness, and anger as they walk past the room they intended to become a nursery.

## Societal expectations of men

Seattle has the reputation of being a place where the yearly rainfall is substantial. But I've visited Seattle on business numerous times, and each visit has been surprisingly sunny. Sure, it rained some during my week-long stays, but overall the weather was beautiful, not anywhere near the gloom and doom advertised. I've joked with my Seattle friends that this rumor must be their way of keeping tourists and potential residents away. They perpetuate the soggy tale just to keep the area to themselves.

Men's struggle with infertility is the opposite of Seattle's reputation. We know infertility is dreary and dark. We know emotional clouds will hang over us frequently, even daily. Yet, when we're with other male friends, even for extended periods of time, we assume a façade. We maintain an outlook that appears sunny, as if infertility were no trouble at all. We behave as if there's no sign of rain in the extended forecast. Sure, a small shower might be mentioned with certain close friends, but on the whole we act like the weather is fine.

Why do men do this? Carol Staudacher, in *Men & Grief*, writes about the cultural expectations of men in today's society. Men are expected to be in control, to be confident, to be more concerned with thinking than feeling, to be rational and analytical, to be assertive, to be courageous and competitive, to accomplish tasks and achieve goals, to be knowledgeable about how mechanical things work, to endure stress without giving up or giving in, to express anger, to be able to bear pain, to be sexually potent, to "settle down" at an appropriate age, to be a devoted husband and father, and to be a provider.

Our society expects a man *not* to lose control over a situation or lose control of himself, to openly cry, to be afraid or anxious, to be dependent, to be passive, to express loneliness or sadness, to express the need for love or affection, to exhibit typically "feminine" characteristics, or to be playful or touch other men.

These opinions pervade our cultural psyche. While there's been some loosening of these expectations in recent times, men are still pressured to live up to them. Anyone caught not doing so is considered less of a man or out of control.

Men's reactions vary radically, but I tend to agree with Staudacher when she says that generally men respond by remaining silent, engaging in solitary mourning or "secret" grief, taking physical or legal action, becoming immersed in activity, and exhibiting addictive behavior.

Men are very good at suppressing their emotions and holding them inside. We learn how to grieve alone. I know a young man whose father died unexpectedly. He kept his emotions out of the public eye by going to his father's grave alone. He never told anyone that this was how he chose to process his grief. His extended family talked often about their absent loved one, so the topic wasn't off-limits. But he wasn't comfortable being part of group grief.

As men, we also process our emotions through activity. Sports give us a safe outlet for shouting at a bad referee call or celebrating a last-second win, whereas venting to God is seen as heresy. We may find refuge at work, where we stay busy with problems and projects that require a different category of emotions, not the painfully personal feelings that swamp our home life. We feel the need to retain some degree of control in most matters, so we find ways to take action physically or legally. We're masters at masking our fears. Typically most men never admit to being afraid of anything. We may be scared out of our minds, but to admit such would be seen as a sign of weakness.

We're taught to be strong. I can't begin to count the number of dramas I've seen that portray a young boy being told, "You're the man of the house now. Be strong for your mother." As husbands, we're tasked with supporting our wives during this time, not ourselves. I was feeling my own sense of anguish, yet I felt the pressure to try to comfort Cindy. I felt I couldn't express my feelings to her since I'm the comforter here, right? Yes, we are comforters for our wives, but I believe there is a need for both—being the comforter and being comforted ourselves.

### Supporting your wife versus supporting yourself

We males are brought up to be the protectors of the family. I would do anything for my wife, up to and including dying for her. With that as my underlying theme, I give every ounce of emotional, physical, mental, and spiritual strength toward supporting her in a time of trial.

You feel the same way about the woman you love. This isn't inherently bad; in fact, your commitment honors God. But as time goes on in your infertility journey, looking out only for her emotional needs ignores your own need for support. If you're making her emotions *the* priority in your life, you're neglecting yours. If you don't get enough self-support, you can't support your wife to the fullest of your ability.

It's not an either/or situation—support her or support yourself. Both of you have valid needs that deserve to be acknowledged. Strive for a balance. There will be days when her needs are most important, and there will be days when your feelings are most important.

Take time for yourself. Weariness will set in if you focus on your wife so completely that you don't take time to recharge your own emotional batteries. Self-support is ever so important if you are to be effective at supporting others. You can't support your wife if you're ignoring or denying your own pain. You and your wife won't self-destruct or fall apart if you're both grieving at the same time and place. We often think, "One of us has to be strong," but this simply is not true.

Men are culturally pressured to be an emotional silo, those massive hollow tanks that store grain. But even silos have a storage limit. Too many men try to hold in all their emotions until they explode one day, maybe uncontrollably. In the same way that the grain has to be released in order to be useful and beneficial to others, a man's emotions need to be released. God's plan is not that men be silos. In His loving wisdom, He created men to be relational beings.

## Lack of male kinship

As infertility dragged on, my heart yearned to share my feelings with an understanding peer, another man who had either been where I was or one who was on the infertility roller coaster himself. I had experienced this type of mutual support during my training days as a chaplain, but now I couldn't find the same type of safe haven to express my sense of utter loss, my anger, my grief, and the frustration that swirled around like a hurricane in my soul.

In general, men experiencing grief lack kinship with peers. We don't have nearly the same support system with other men that women have with one another.

A prime example of this showed up as we researched this book by surveying couples via mail and email. There was little or no response from the husbands on the returned questionnaires. Several wives said they couldn't get their husbands to sit down to answer the questions. More than one woman said her husband didn't want to think back and try to recall his feelings during infertility. One woman even stated that the husband perceived the problem was only with the wife's reproductive organs, so he felt he had nothing to contribute to the survey. Was he totally oblivious to the infertility struggle his wife faced? Probably not, but he denied his emotional ownership in the problem.

I'd venture that men's lack of input on our questionnaire has to do not only with the lack of willingness to share emotions but with the inability to name our emotions in the first place, to identify what we're feeling, and to face the depth of those emotions.

One couple we hoped would share their opinions simply never responded. Though I saw the couple almost weekly and thought the infertility battle was fresh on their minds, they kept putting it off. "We're working on it," was their typical response; and after numerous requests, I just stopped asking. Finally, the wife told me that her husband couldn't fill out the survey because it was "too painful" for him. They were deep in the throes of infertility treatments, and neither wanted to share that pain because it was just too hard. If the pain of scribbling words on an innocuous piece of paper is too much to handle, how much harder will it be for a flesh-and-blood person to live through?

For a man, a deep friendship with another man will bring the benefits of both sharing emotions and practical assistance. I sincerely believe that we, as men, need to foster a relationship with another man who knows about the storms of infertility. And either now or later, we can provide a safe haven for another man by being his friend in the midst of his personal storm.

When I experienced the joy of being able to share my emotions with a group of peers in a safe place, I let go of heartaches that were weighing so heavily on me at the time. There is no experience like being able to bare your soul and let others support you. They didn't have all the answers, but there's a certain amount of cleansing that occurs simply by opening up.

I have also experienced a time where I desperately needed and wanted to share, but found no avenue to do so. This was one of the darkest periods of my life. I had tasted water from the well of sharing and I knew what it was like, but my wilderness during this time was dry and dusty. How my heart longed to drink from that well again, but no oasis could be found. I made it through that wilderness, but it was one of the hardest trials of my life.

**How to begin talking about your feelings**
I am confident that communication of our emotions is the right thing to do. Having the ability to become comfortable sharing these deep emotions with others is no easy undertaking. As with any major skill in our lives, it takes practice. For

anyone to be able to share deep feelings with another person, he has to share feelings often. Men aren't in the habit of doing that.

Because women have grown up sharing in this way from childhood, they have more practice and experience. Men can learn some things from this. First, we see that it can be done. Second, it helps to be able to express these emotions out loud. Third, we can find a safe place or support group to share with. Fourth, we needn't be afraid to try.

Take the chance to open up your silo of feelings with someone you know, and work hard to continue to share those feelings. Once you do it, you will begin to reap the benefits of sharing as you gain confidence and comfort. Make every effort to share, but be patient with yourself. It is a learned experience and trust has to be established and built. And who better to share with than someone who has had a parallel journey? Ask around your church and other areas in your life. You'll be surprised at the number of people you will hear about who know firsthand of infertility or adoption. Take that first step. You will not be disappointed.

## Naming and identifying your emotions

When I was a chaplain at a large hospital in Alabama, my supervisor taught me and my fellow chaplains a great skill at being able to name our feelings. She would ask us during some of our interpersonal relationship seminars to express how a situation made us feel. We would launch into a discussion, rambling around the feeling and not really naming it. Finally, she would halt our dialogue and hold up her hand with her fingers spread apart. "These are your options," she'd say as she pointed to each finger to emphasize each choice, "Mad, Sad, Glad, Scared, or Hurt. You have to use one of these to define your feelings. No other words are acceptable."

We were forced to use only those five words to label what we had been rambling about. The other words we used to dance around the topic weren't tolerated. And when one of us would venture back into talking around our feelings without really pinpointing them, she would just hold up her hand again and point. It was an action she repeated so often that she didn't even need to speak. Just the action of her pointing toward her outstretched palm was enough for us to rethink what we were saying and give it a name.

This exercise pushed us to identify our emotions within specific categories, rather than verbose descriptions that sometimes revealed nothing. It helped us to name our emotions and led us to talk about them aloud with someone who understood what we were saying. We all had common ground in understanding what the terms meant.

### Loss of dreams for fatherhood

Have you dreamed of playing catch with your son, hearing the snap of the glove around a white baseball with tight, red laces? Or, maybe you envision tossing a 165-gram regulation Frisbee on the beach. A myriad of dreams for how you'll interact with your son . . . now appear to be slipping away.

And you have hopes and dreams for your daughter as well. Teaching her to ride a bike and hoping beyond hope she doesn't fall too hard. Terrorizing her first suitor when he picks her up for a date. A hopeful father's countless dreams for his daughter are dashed in the midst of infertility struggles.

Men, as well as women, have hopes for their future children. Our dreams often go unspoken, or at least, they're not spoken of as freely as the dreams of women. We have dreams about what our children will one day become. We find ourselves thinking of these things even more when the future looks dark surrounding our potential fatherhood.

*After a few months of struggle, the reality starts to settle in and our hopes for our children come crashing down around our feet like the autumn leaves falling from an ancient oak tree. They lie there and wait for someone to pick them up, but mostly people walk through and kick them out of the path. Try as we might, it's impossible to put these leaves back on the tree. There is a deep, cold winter that blows in and strips every last leaf off the tree. Like the tree in spring, though, our hopes can be renewed as we move into the next season. But during autumn and winter, spring seems so far away, and the nights are so long, it feels like they will last an eternity.*

*—my journal*

### The anguish of an empty room

When do you decorate a nursery if there's no expected due

date? For years we envisioned turning a room into a nursery, filling it with our collection of Pooh Bears, decorating walls and bedding in that "bear of very little brain" theme. We just had no idea *when* that might be. It was a room for which we had plans and decorations. It was a room we couldn't bring ourselves to decorate until we were closer to completing either a successful pregnancy or adoption. The room tangibly symbolized that we were "without child." I could feel my anguish rise when I walked into the room. I ached so for a child, for Cindy as well as for myself. "Where's the nursery?" kept echoing in my head.

My advice? Don't decorate a nursery until you're well on your way to an adoption or a successful pregnancy. Even if it's not all finished when you bring a baby home, you can find time to get the most important things done. Adoptive couples sometimes have little warning that a child is coming their way, but more than once, I've seen God provide the goods for these hastily assembled nurseries. Our adoption of Ryan was so accelerated that we had only four days between learning he would be ours until he was placed in our arms. We didn't even have time to find a baby bed. God's provision came through when Ryan's birth mother gave us all the nursery items she received when she thought she was going to keep her baby—bassinet, car seat, two strollers, boxes of clothes, diapers, toys, bedding. We had an instant nursery the day Ryan arrived home.

## Will my name die out with me?

When my paternal grandfather passed away in 1987 while I was attending seminary, I fully realized that I was the last male to carry on the Dake name. My own father was still living, but it was evident at my grandfather's death that it fell to me to continue the name of my forefathers.

You may be the last male in a long bloodline and facing the same fear. The older we get and the longer it takes for conception or adoption to occur, the more this fear is realized.

Some families may imply that passing along your name to an adopted child isn't quite "official" enough. This gets tricky emotionally because you're pulled between the joy of finally becoming a father and the anger/hurt that some relatives may not accept your adopted child as a valid recipient of the name since there's no blood relation.

Talk with your wife about your fears and feelings on this issue. Talk with your parents or other relatives who you believe would be supportive of your choice to adopt, if that's what you decide to do. In other words, rally some moral support for your case before sitting down with anyone who doesn't feel the same sense of acceptance. If you and your wife believe in your hearts that God has led you to build your family through adoption, then rest in that truth. God will speak to *you and your wife* about how to build *your* family; He won't give the instructions to your grandparents.

It helps to remember that God's Word is very clear on the truth that He has adopted each believer as His own (Rom. 8:15; Eph. 1:5). When relatives get hung up on the need for offspring to come only via the bloodline, they are denying the validity of the adoptive relationship God has initiated with each person who chooses to have a personal relationship with Jesus Christ.

### Is something wrong with me?
Guilt, fear, and embarrassment. That's what this question brings to mind. The fear is always there for the male that there may be something wrong with you or your body.

*The actual emotions were obviously a sense of failure, inadequacy, and being somewhat less than a man. However, that rational side of being a man took over and simply steered my focus to solving the problem. It was very eye-opening to see the harsh reality and almost coldness of diagnosing and treating infertility. You are poked, prodded, tested, and thoroughly examined. Not that my physician was uncaring or insensitive, but there are only so many ways that you can perform the medical work-up necessary, and yet maintain some amount of dignity and modesty in the process.* —Jim

Women often say these very same feelings overwhelm them and, considering the endless procedures a woman endures, she has a right to feel that way. But men also experience it in varying degrees. It's especially true at the start of the infertility journey until the diagnosis is made, if the source of the problem can be identified at all. Unless a man gets the "all clear" signal from the doctor, indicating that his half of the reproductive process is working well, a man will have this nagging sense of failure and inadequacy all the way through.

*Tests determined that I had sperm antibodies. I felt like I was the main reason that we had to do ICSI. I felt like my body was letting us down. This was hard to swallow. It hurt my ego.* —Greg

Guilt is the constant companion of fear in this reality. A man can feel guilty for having an infertility problem that keeps them from realizing their dreams of having a child. "It's my fault," we say to ourselves again and again. "There has to be *something* we can do to can fix the problem so I can give my wife the object of her dreams." But with male factor infertility, the options are limited. Our drive to *do something* runs us right into a brick wall.

Frustration abounds. If your body is the major infertility issue, then there will be times that you will be angry with yourself. There will be times that the emotions will be so overwhelming that you may say inappropriate things to family, friends, and especially to your wife. Then you've added even more guilt and frustration to your already heavy load.

These feelings all comprise the kind of situation that needs to be expressed to another man. Find someone to share these feelings with so your anger can be released in a timely and appropriate way. Don't allow it to eat away at you from the inside, undermining your spiritual and emotional foundation until you feel as if your life is about to fall in on itself.

## Protecting your wife from pain and suffering

Men want to protect their wives from the pain and suffering during infertility. Yet, you may be required to give your wife an injection every day as part of a treatment. This experience can be extremely painful for your wife, and actively participating in the administration of such discomfort can be agonizing for you too.

You know that these injections have to be given to create the opportunity to possibly conceive. You know it's the doctor's orders that you give these meds to your wife. But it's hard to logically and mentally realize those things when emotionally you're causing her extreme physical pain simply by doing what you're supposed to do. The result is an internal wrestling match between your heart and mind. Sometimes the mind wins this daily match, and it's easier to understand the need for the injections, and thus the pain. Other times, the heart pins the mind to the mat, making it harder to bring yourself to continue.

*I just hurt so much for Dinah because she endured physically much more than I did. Her tests were more extensive. She was the one having surgery and taking multiple medications that produced such difficult side effects. I loved her and didn't like to see her hurting so.*
*—Keith*

This is a breeding ground for frustration and anger within you. You'll make attempts to shield your wife from the hurt of another failed conception—like trying to convince her it's time to stop pursuing biological children altogether. You may downplay your own emotions to protect her from feeling so disappointed when failure strikes again. Be prepared for the fact that she may not respond well to your attempts because they seem to counter her goal—conception no matter the cost.

The old saying goes: "There's no anger like a woman scorned." To create a parallel proverb, we might say: "There's no frustration like a man who tries to protect his wife, but to no avail." Share your frustration with your wife. Let her know that you hurt when you have to give her injections. Let her know the struggle going on in your soul as you participate in this required regimen.

Get some opinions from other men who have had to do the same thing. With so many couples pursuing infertility that require at-home injections, you'll find their insights comforting, if for no other reason than that they to confirm that you're not alone.

### A necessary evil: sperm samples
Infertility procedures make it necessary to harvest the male contribution to the fertilization process. This sometimes involves going to a physician's office or a special collection

center to donate sperm before the eggs are ready to receive the sperm, depending on which alphabetical formula is required for possible conception—IVF, ICSI, GIFT, ZIFT, and so forth.

For many males, this is a mind-numbing experience in which the embarrassment is well beyond the normal limits. The full force of the embarrassment is unleashed when you arrive at the office and the reality hits you that everyone you talk to in an official capacity knows exactly why you're there. No one overtly speaks about it, but covertly we're hypersensitive, knowing that they all know. And they know we know they know! It's as though everyone is somewhat embarrassed by the situation, and this makes it even more embarrassing for you. This can be one of the toughest acts to participate in for the man during this trying time.

If there were a way we could bottle up this embarrassment and sell it, it would have a far greater effect on dampening sexual excitement than the proverbial cold shower. Coupled with the embarrassment is the fact that, because of the embarrassment, the activity takes longer. Because it takes longer, it becomes even more embarrassing. And so the cycle goes.

I remember the instruction sheet that was given to us when they wanted to do some tests on all the attributes of my semen. A little collection cup and a test tube were provided. Thankfully, we could collect the sample at home. "It has to be brought to the office within an hour after collection," the instructions stated. "Keep the specimen warm. Make sure to get as much of the specimen in the test tube as you can." Easy for *them* to say!

We decided on a morning donation. This is a unique situation for husbands and wives. Although Cindy tried to lessen my anxiety, I knew what was required. The whole idea of producing a specimen for a test tube has the result of putting a damper on any semblance of arousal that might have been possible should this have been any other time. Then, the sheer fact that this very personal specimen is going to a lab for evaluation and diagnosis is beyond being a nonaphrodisiac. I tried not to let my imagination run away, but it's easy to feel that your very manhood is on the line, about to be defined for better or worse in terms related to motility, density, and how many millions you can produce.

I finally succeeded in acquiring a sample, which led to an additional form of embarrassment for Cindy. In order to keep the semen warm, she followed the suggestions given to her by placing the test tube next to her skin, held in place by her skirt waistband. This was fine until she got into the car to head to the physician's office in the strictly allotted time. When the automatic seat belt moved into position, she noticed a problem. The seat belt came right over the top of the test tube and pressed it firmly against her skin. Driving to the downtown clinic, she had visions of having a fender bender on the way. What if the test tube shattered from the impact? What if the glass punctured her skin? What if she bled pro-fusely, and the officer who responded asked if she was hurt? How embarrassing would it be to explain that a test tube of semen had caused her injury! Fortunately, she made it safely to the doctor's office and delivered the warm sample within the time allotted.

I can't speak for females in the similar act of preparing, sonograming, and harvesting their eggs, but I'm sure they have parallel feelings regarding some of these procedures. Tell your wife how it makes you feel. Let her explain how her pro-cedures affect her. Sharing your experiences, even the embar-rassing ones, will help you connect during this part of the journey.

## Enduring waiting rooms and embarrassing silences

There is nothing worse to me than having to discuss very inti-mate topics with complete strangers. Sometimes it's easier because you may never see a nurse again, but these never-see-you-again people are rare in the field of infertility. The med-ical personnel at the clinic quickly come to know you as a couple, but in the initial meeting these people are typically complete strangers. It seems not to faze them when they start asking very confidential questions and discussing private acts and situations.

But even before you get to the room in the inner office, you have to endure the waiting room. As I saw other men in the waiting room with their wives, I found myself wondering, "What are they thinking about me?" Then it hit me: *They're*

*probably thinking the same thing I am, and wondering what every-*
*one is thinking about them.* So all of us were sitting there feeling
equally insecure and embarrassed.

So how do you handle those embarrassing silences? Don't
let it paralyze you. Acknowledge it, but don't give in to its
siren song. It beckons you to give in and run far away. Fight
or flight? Everything in me wanted to choose flight! Utilize
your willpower and push through the overwhelming feelings
until you reach the goal of having your named to follow the
nurse to an examination room.

## Expressing your anger

It's okay to grieve. It's okay to be angry. It's okay to express to
God that sense of betrayal. Find a safe place where you can
express these feelings. It may be with your spouse or it may
be with a close male friend, but find that place. This will give
you a needed release and move you closer to supporting others when it's time for you to provide that support.

In the movie *Shadowlands,* the character of C. S. Lewis says,
"I pray because I can't help myself. I pray because I'm helpless. I pray because the need flows out of me all the time,
waking and sleeping. It doesn't change God. It changes me."

My journey of grief and pain has taught me a number of
things, but most important, it has taught me that prayer is
important. Just as vital as it is to share your hurt with your
wife and let her share hers with you, so you must share your
feelings with God.

I remember days, weeks, even months that seemed like the
darkest times I had ever endured in my life. I felt there was
no hope of light breaking through. My head knew that God
was in control. My experience told me that God had been
faithful in past dark moments in my life. But my heart often
seemed to win the battle, telling me that there was no hope
for a solution. I found myself very angry with God. The injustice of the situation ignited my anger at Him. We're good people who have so much love to give to a child. Why doesn't
God allow us a child?

This anger wasn't easy to share with people. Most people
had a hard time allowing me to be angry with God. They
would tell me not to feel that way. They would try to defend

God. I see no need for any human to defend God from the impact of my emotions. My faith is such that I believe God is quite capable of defending Himself. I also take solace in the fact that the people in the Bible who had a close relationship with God were the ones who could express their anger to Him. The many psalms David penned display his blunt honesty before God. And think of the journeys experienced by Jeremiah, Habakkuk, Job, Moses, Gideon, Peter, Mary, Martha, Jonah, Elijah, and Jesus. Even the martyred saints in heaven question God's delay of judgment and avenging their blood (Rev. 6:10).

The safest place I had to express that anger was directly to God. He was not crushed by it. He wasn't offended by it. He knew it was there, so why even hold it back? I found it cleansing and freeing to share my anger with Him. He could be trusted with my deepest, even ugliest, emotions. There are times that I longed to share it with a man, a peer, who would understand; but, sadly, I was never able to find anyone who could handle hearing my deepest emotions.

To be honest, there will be times when you'll be angry with your wife. The stress of infertility holds both of you in a vise grip, making your emotional fuse shorter, your anger more likely to erupt than under normal circumstances.

Then there was my anger at society at large—abandoned children, unwanted children, abused children, aborted children. I hurt so much when I thought of all these little lives lost or in crisis that eventually the hurt turned into anger toward a culture that lets it happen. The abortion rate stabbed my heart—in an average year 1.3 million babies are aborted with a total of more than 38 million since 1973. Cindy and I couldn't even achieve one solitary pregnancy, yet all these babies were, in our opinion, murdered.

Allow yourself the freedom to feel the emotion of anger. Our society has no problem with men showing their anger, but you must not let it be the only emotion you express or share. Remember: Mad, Glad, Sad, Scared, or Hurt.

And how do you usually express anger? Do you shout at the nearest person who happens to trip your switch? Do you throw something? There are healthier ways to vent your anger—exercise is a great one. Almost any kind of exercise will do. Go for a jog or very intense walk. Find a punching bag at the gym. Get on a bike and pedal away your angst. Push a lawn mower around the yard at record speeds. Chop some firewood for next winter. Give yourself the freedom to try different venues to express your anger so that you don't take it out on a person.

## A quest for answers

You will have countless questions during your journey, questions that don't have answers—at least not acceptable ones. The infertility experience will rock your faith to its foundation. There will be times of weeping. There will be times of mourning. There may be times of death—miscarriage, stillbirth, failed adoption. Ecclesiastes states that there is a time for everything under the sun. We must allow ourselves the freedom to experience, acknowledge, and process the pains.

I wonder sometimes if the questions one has in the darkest moments of infertility will ever see the light of day. Could it be that these questions that plague countless infertile couples maintain their existence in the dark? John Claypool, a minister whose young daughter died of leukemia, states it so eloquently in his *Tracks of a Fellow Struggler*:

*I have found no answers to the deepest questions of this experience. When I first heard the diagnosis and went out alone to cry, I asked the same things anyone would ask: "Why has this happened? Why do little girls get leukemia? Why is there leukemia at all? Why is there sickness and suffering and pain in a world that is supposed to be the creation of an all-good and all-powerful God? . . . I found no neat and tidy answers to lay them to rest. . . . Up to this moment, nowhere have I found any single answer that settles all the questions or accounts for all the nuances of this tragic occurrence. The enigma remains what it has been from the beginning—a dark mystery for which there is no satisfactory explanation.*

He goes on to explain that his faith challenged him to go on living "even though I have no answer or any complete explanation." Another thing of "tremendous value" was that the Bible and his faith gave him "a stern warning to beware of superficiality and quick labeling, of jumping to the wrong conclusions. If the Bible says anything to us about life, it is that this existence of ours is a deep and complex and mysterious affair."

The key is that we learn to live with these unanswerable questions, to coexist with them. We may never find the answers to these questions. We may move well beyond our infertility struggle and even be blessed with a child, but these questions could remain unanswered for the length of our days.

In the years to come, other people will come to you looking for answers as they walk their paths of grief. As you learn to live without completely understanding your tragic experiences, you will one day be able to help others find peace with the "deepest questions" and "darkest mysteries."

## A message for wives

While at times it may feel that you—the one trying to carry a baby in your body—are alone in this infertility battle, remember that you are assuredly not alone. You have a partner in this wilderness journey. Your husband is there with you and walking alongside you in your seemingly endless wanderings through choices, decisions, pain, and frustration.

He may not be able to adequately express his feelings to you in the manner that you're craving, but know that he is hurting and aching for your hurt to be removed. Help him help you by letting him know what you need. Help him name and express some of his feelings so that you can both discuss them on common ground. Familiarize yourself with the Mad, Glad, Sad, Scared, Hurt exercise. Allow your husband to explain his feelings in a manner that helps you understand the depth of his emotions.

Most important, don't place your own feelings of what he is trying to say upon his statements. Allow his words to be his. Don't assume that you know what he means, just because you know what it means to you. Let him tell you what it means to him.

Be comfortable with silence when asking your husband for an answer to a question or to name a feeling. He is processing something that may be new to him and it may take some time to come up with an answer.

Your husband feels a dire need to protect you from your pain. There are some tangible ways he may show this. He might express anger at family members who say inappropriate things regarding the inability to conceive quickly. He may show a lack of interest or avoid church during Mother's Day, Father's Day, or other holidays. He may not encourage participation in social gatherings that involve other couples.

He may express his anger in ways that don't seem appropriate. Be understanding; help him to identify the reason for his misdirected anger. Ask leading questions that help him identify what his anger arises from, and where or at whom his anger is directed. Encourage him to discover new ways to vent his anger appropriately.

Know that your husband loves you. You may feel unlovable or even unloved during this time. Godly husbands care for their wives deeply and, during infertility, hurt with them as only a partner of one flesh can hurt. His love for you is deep and strong. Ask him to share this love on the days when you need to feel it the most and accept it on days when he needs to express it to you.

You are both in the midst of a raging storm. You are both experiencing most of the same emotions. You both express these emotions, but in different ways. Join with each other and hold tightly to God. In this way you can help your husband grow closer to God when he's feeling abandoned, and he can do the same for you.

Your journey is a long road, and the end may not be in sight. Expect storms and rain. Anticipate times when one of you will start to slip. Help each other to stay the course. In doing so, your troubles will be halved and your joys will be doubled. This is my earnest prayer for you both.

*Joe and Julie*

# The best thing and the worst thing

Joe and Julie's first date was at a youth banquet where he was leading music. The speaker talked about facing your greatest fear. Afterwards, Joe asked Julie what her greatest fear was.

Without missing a beat, Julie said, "My greatest fear is that I would never be able to have children, that I would never be a mom." Reality has a way of calling us back to poignant moments from our past, and that moment would haunt Joe again and again.

After they were married, they eventually began trying to get pregnant—unsuccessfully. "I kept remembering Julie's remark, and it terrified me," he said. Initial testing revealed Julie was fine, but Joe had several male factor infertility issues. As the doctor told Joe over the phone that he was the cause of their infertility, Joe remembers, "In a moment, my whole manhood, my whole sense of worth was sucked down the drain. I started bawling. I told Julie, 'I am your fear come true.' Nothing can be more humiliating for a man. I almost went off the deep end."

They were given a 1-in-800 chance of becoming pregnant. Infertility treatments were not even attempted. Then, seven years into their infertility, on what they call Black Monday, they were told Joe's sperm count was below one million and that it would be impossible for them to ever have children.

"But nine months to the day from Black Monday, we adopted Samuel. Even in our grief, God was preparing for us to adopt. It was the biggest thrill of our lives," Joe said. "The moment they laid Samuel in our arms, he was our child. Our fear with adoption was, could we ever love somebody else's child like we would love our own? Well, with an adoption under our belts, our biggest fear was whether we could ever love biological children as we love our adopted son!"

Their adoption was subject to the laws of the state where Samuel was born. Those laws gave the birth parents forty days to change their minds, plus another ten days to state why they hadn't made it to court in forty days. On day forty-two, Samuel's birth father made known his wishes to reclaim his son. The birth mother didn't change her mind.

Joe and Julie found themselves in a tiny category of parents whose adoptions are contested by a birth parent (only one-tenth of 1 percent [0.1]). A court hearing, expected to last two or three days, was scheduled. Joe and Julie tried to prepare themselves for the horrible possibility of losing their son.

Joe describes the worst day of his life as the Sunday before the Monday hearing was to begin. As a pastor, Joe was prepared to preach the three morning services that Sunday. Julie had stayed home with Samuel. Joe listened as a soloist sang about trusting God implicitly—when you can't trace His hand, trust His heart.

"I walked up to the pulpit, but I was so upset I couldn't see my notes. I didn't want to be there. I just walked out. To this day, I don't know what they did in those three services." (Unbeknownst to Joe, I called his church and asked the staff what happened. I learned that during those services, the church family spent time praying for Joe, Julie, and Samuel.)

"I went home and mowed the lawn for the fourth time that weekend. I always mowed around one particular sprinkler head; but at that moment, I decided to just shear it off to give myself something to do."

He went to the hardware store for a new sprinkler head and saw Jim, an employee, assembling a child's bicycle. Jim was complaining about the complexities of putting together a bike, and he said, "Can you think of any good reason to put a bike together?"

Joe remembers that very moment as "the absolute lowest moment of my life. I had one dream at that time: I wanted to build a bike for my son. I didn't care about growing a church. I didn't even care about my role as a husband at that moment. I just wanted the chance to build a bike for my son. I thought, 'If I lose that boy, I don't think I'll be able to make it.'"

"That worst day of my life was followed by the very best day of my life. On Monday, the judge had awarded Samuel to us." What was supposed to have been a three-day trial was over in just a few hours. The birth father had shown up in court late, drunk, and without any proof of his ability to parent a child. The judge decided that Samuel's best interests were served with Joe and Julie.

All that was left was for Joe and Julie and Samuel to travel to his birth state and sign the documents officially finalizing the adoption. It was a huge ordeal, as both sides of their extended families came to the hearing, scheduled to take place in the judge's private chambers because the courtroom was being repainted.

"I had earlier asked our lawyer if he knew of anything that could go wrong. This was supposed to be an open-and-shut thing. He jokingly said, 'Well, a plane could crash into the building, or you could have a heart attack.' We had just shaken hands with the judge to begin the hearing when we were told there was a bomb threat and the entire building was being evacuated." Exiting the building, the lawyer looked at Joe and said, " . . . Or a bomb threat!"

Standing on the parking lot with the crowd of other evacuees, the judge agreed to hear the case if a stenographer could be found; but one couldn't be located. For a while, it looked as if they would have to postpone their hearing for another six months. Then suddenly it was announced they could return to the building. The hearing took place as planned, finally.

Joe, Julie, and Samuel settled into a normal routine after that. But one day Joe was asked to come to the ob/gyn's office to be with Julie during a sonogram. A test had come back with questionable results and there was a fear of ovarian cancer.

While watching the sonogram the doctor sounded surprised: "Well, what do we have here?"

Joe and Julie were pregnant. Luke was born, and then Joe had reparative surgery. Two years later, Hannah was born; followed by Grace a few years later.

"We love all our kids so much, but adoption is ten times the trip that a birth ever was! Infertility was the worst thing that ever happened to us, and it was the best thing that ever happened to us. Without it, we would never have adopted Samuel. And if God had not been the foundation of our home, infertility would have been the storm that removed our home from its foundation."

Chapter 4

# *Marriage—Will Yours Survive or Thrive?*

*We became closer, mostly because of Keith's efforts. There were many times that I would just kind of "check out" and not want to talk or face the issue, but Keith would not let it pass. He was my strength and my hero through it all! We are very close and have been blessed with a relationship that I only dreamed about before.*

*—Dinah*

A co-worker who has three children sat near me at lunch one day. Munching on our sandwiches, from out of nowhere he asked me if my husband and I were going to have children. I told him that I thought we would probably start a family in the next few years, but I wasn't sure. "Why else would you get married?" he asked incredulously. Then he went on to spout his opinion that marriage was for the purpose of producing children. I just kept chewing and offering a thoughtful "hmmm" once in a while. I could think of plenty of reasons to disagree with him, but I was sure the resulting discussion would give me indigestion.

Some people get married to have children, but most of us realize that marriage is not just a means to that particular end. Marriage for the sole purpose of bearing children misses out on all that is wonderful and unique in a union planned by the Creator Himself.

Marriage is such an incredible partnership when you think about it. God created this concept of a permanent union between a man and woman, a union that would make each stronger than they could be separately. Best friends united for life. The minister at our wedding, Roy Fish, called it "God's mathematics." He explained that marriage means sharing both joys and sorrows, and that in sharing both the ups and downs of life, a couple's joys are doubled and their sorrows are halved.

I've always liked that last statement especially: joys doubled, sorrows halved. But when the sorrow is infertility, even half a sorrow weighs a whale of a lot more than you expect. When both partners are limping along emotionally from infertility's pain, the emotional baggage is a ten-ton weight. How can a marriage endure under that kind of strain? How can a wife and husband stay sane through the trials, tests, and endless diagnostic measures? How can your love survive and thrive so that when a child enters your life, your marriage is equipped to take on the added pressures of parenthood?

**How can he or she not understand what I'm feeling?**
Husbands and wives misread each other for some very elemental reasons, succinctly stated in two words: *estrogen* and *testosterone.* The implications are complicated, but the foundations are pretty simple.

Estrogen and testosterone are the hormones that flood our respective systems from our time in the womb. They are what make us uniquely female and male, what make us fit together so wonderfully, and what pit us against each other so frustratingly. Testosterone makes men generally have less need to exercise the verbal portions of their brains. It makes them content with segmenting life into compartments that can be brought out one at a time to consider and interact with. On the flip side, estrogen gives women the capacity to verbalize about twice as much as men each day, describing events and experiences with incredible (or exhausting) detail. It enables them to see their lives, not in compartments, but as one big continuum.

Men don't understand women's overflowing feelings, and women don't understand men's understated emotions. However, it's not a great divide with no bridge. As adults who love each other, you can build a bridge of communication across the chasm.

I consider my husband to be rather atypical on the male scale, but he's still more cautious with his word volume than I am. One of his qualities that first appealed to me was that he wrote poetry—wow! A man in touch with his ability to use words creatively! When we began brainstorming this book, we decided that Edward would write the chapter on how men feel during infertility experiences. I told him to aim for 4,000 words. But his first draft, which seemed complete to him, hit only 2,300 words. I looked through his material, noted a half-dozen areas for him to expound on, and several weeks later he gave me his finished rough draft—11,223 words! I nearly fainted. At 2,300 words, he'd thought he didn't have anything more to say.

Men can be lovingly encouraged to get in touch with their emotions and their abilities to express them. If you're expecting your husband to one day be as voluntarily expressive as you are, well, don't hang your hat on that dream. Your goal is that you are aware of each other's feelings, that you are communicating on an emotional level during one of the most trying stages of your marriage.

Make it a point to sit down with each other at regular checkpoints during your infertility journey and hear each other's feelings on where you've been, where you are, and where you might be headed. Talk about the next stage of treatments that are being considered. Keep an open mind about reworking your plans based on what you hear your spouse say about how he or she is thinking and feeling.

Ladies, once you get your man talking, you might need to hone your listening skills. We're the ones who fill in the ends of sentences, put words in their mouths, and jump in to tell them what *we* think. Listen as if you will need to give a detailed verbal summary when he finishes. Listen like you'd like to be listened to.

### Anger, blame, and other ugly things

This almost goes without saying, but there will be times when you're angry at your spouse. And there will be times when he or she is angry at you.

The world (or your marriage) won't fall apart because you blew up at each other. After the dust clears, sit down with each other and talk about *why* (yes, that three-letter word) you got angry. Look inside yourself and identify what made you mad, sad, glad, scared, hurt to the point that it resulted in anger. Anger as a response isn't always caused by an anger-inducing stimulus. Sometimes anger is what happens after a hurt has gone untended for too long or a fear has simmered under the surface.

*Every time my period came along, I was really bummed out. I'd mention it to my husband and he would almost always say something like, "We'll just keep trying, Sweetie." Maybe he was a little too perky, too upbeat; but whatever he did, it wasn't really the response I was looking for. One day, I jumped down his throat and yelled, "But I don't want to just keep trying!" Honestly, I don't know what response I was hoping for. Probably nothing would really be an effective comfort.*
                                                                    —Lou Ann

Besides aiming anger at each other, we get angry at ourselves because our bodies aren't working right. An infertile woman feels that her body has let her down. For thousands of years, women have birthed children as regularly as the seasons change. Did I mar my fertility by something I did? Or is it spiritual punishment for a past mistake? An infertile man faces similar questions with unique implications. Was it a sports injury? Was it reckless behavior?

The "broken" partner can muster up a truckload of guilt or may feel that his or her spouse is blaming him or her, even though the spouse is unaware of this perception. *In trying to identify the reason you are infertile, you are trying to find the bad guy.*

When a crime has been committed, society searches for the criminal, never wanting to settle for an unsolved crime. With infertility, finding the bad guy (the cause) helps you deal with grief because you can aim all those bad feelings at a target. Once you find the problem, then you have to figure how to deal with it. But if your fertility problems remain a mystery, and many do, you have to live with never knowing why you can't conceive. No bad guy, nowhere to aim the blame.

**Effects on your marriage**
No one really expects that infertility will knock on their front door. But when it does, you're totally blown away by the pain

it brings to your marriage. Ann and Wallace had friends who had been unsuccessful after one in vitro fertilization (IVF). "Even though we saw our friends suffering," she said, "we didn't realize the severity of the pain until it was ours." Ann and Wallace struggled through three unsuccessful IVFs before moving on to adoption. Celeste only knew one other couple who had been going through infertility for about three years: "I saw how it totally consumed them. I knew I would never be like that. But I became *exactly* like that."

*Tension? Difficulty? Absolutely! Bob was frustrated by my laid-back "things will work out" attitude. I mourned my childlessness while Bob had a much more task-oriented "what must we do to solve this?" attitude.* —Paula

Marriage resembles a three-legged race. Both partners have one leg free, but the other leg is bound to their spouse. Walking and even trotting is fine as long as both are in sync with each other and the terrain is predictable. But when one spouse hits a bump, the whole partnership is thrown off balance. When one is limping along, the other can't zoom along unaffected. Both slow down to keep from falling flat on their faces. The partnership is only as healthy as the individuals.

And you think it's stressful *now?* Your love needs to survive and thrive so that when a child enters your life, your marriage is equipped to take on the added pressures of parenthood. Most couples run headlong into pregnancy or adoption with little or no time in between the stages of crisis and pending resolution. In other words, if a fertility procedure works and she conceives and carries to term, you have nine months of being totally wrapped up in the anticipated delivery. Then you're thrown into the sleep-deprived world of new parenthood. You don't get to take a few months out to heal your marriage from the stress of your infertile years. If you end up with a baby, but your marriage is falling apart, it's not pleasant for you, it doesn't honor God, and it doesn't do your baby any good either. God wants your marriage to be stronger as a result of the trials you walk through.

Consider these ideas for strengthening your marriage:
1. *Pray together daily.*
2. *Get into God's Word together.*
3. *Be intentional about strengthening your support system with family and friends.*

## Intimacy just ain't what it used to be
One thing is for sure: Infertility takes the fun out of your love life. Everyone agrees on that.

*The drudgery of infertility took its toll on our physical intimacy. Much of the spontaneity was gone and intimacy became very "clinical" as we worried about timing, frequency, hormone levels, etc.*
—*Paula and Bob*

*While we were doing some testing to see who was the "problem," we were both tense, stressed, and disappointed that things weren't happening naturally. Also, when we were charting the ovulation temperatures and keeping track of all that, sex was often a "have to" instead of a "want to." That was strenuous for both of us. We were trying to achieve something, and we just couldn't make it happen.*
—*Deana and Lane*

*We had to have sex on one particular night so that I could be tested the next morning. That evening was horrible. We sat on opposite sides of the house, mad at each other. Sex was the last thing on our minds.*                                                      —*Beth and Brian*

Spontaneity is what brings vitality to your love life. A schedule, a timetable, and a temperature chart all throw cold water on spontaneity. But you can fight back with some intentional "mind games," and some understanding along the way.

## Accept the fact that there will be times when you have sex for functional reasons only.
Just being mentally prepared for those times can help you take it a little more in stride. Mentally separate clinical intercourse from marital intimacy. In other words, go through the motions when you have to, but give yourselves a rain check for an enjoyable session together at another time.

### Revive the courtship.
Do you still go on dates together, or do you just rush out for a bite to eat and maybe catch a movie? Treat each other as special, like when you were first dating. Husband, call your wife from work and ask her out on an official date. Dress up. Bring her a flower. Keep romance alive by feeding it something new once in a while. Revisit the places you went on your first dates.

### Consider a weekend away.
You may be pinching pennies these days to pay for fertility treatments, but once in a blue moon, go away for a weekend together. Change your scenery for a while and breathe some fresh air. Remember, these weekend escapes will be harder to come by once a baby enters your life. Grab the moments while you can.

Two days after we got the news that I didn't qualify for a fertility study group (which was our last hope for fertility treatments), Edward and I both took a Friday off and designated it as our play day. We went out for breakfast—peach-covered pancakes—then we saw two movies in a row. Midafternoon, we indulged in cream-filled doughnuts, then went to the mall for some just-because-we-want-to shopping. It was a fun, responsibility-less day that helped to balance out the tough news we'd received that week.

### Feelings, emotions, and opinions
To borrow from the old Yellow Pages theme song, spouses who "reach out and touch" on multiple levels have marriages that survive and thrive through infertility. A husband knows his wife physically needs a warm hug after she hangs up from talking with the fertility clinic. She knows how to touch him on an emotional/mental level by reading his behavior. He touches her heart spiritually when she hears him praying for their relationship to grow stronger in spite of this difficulty.

Staying tuned in to each other on these various levels requires determination and intentionality. It doesn't just happen. But if you don't *work* to stay in touch, then your marriage will be on shaky ground before you ever reach the delivery room.

Make an effort to understand your spouse's emotions throughout your infertility journey. Don't assume you know how she feels when she has to attend her friend's baby shower. Don't try to guess how he's handling the next stage of treatments. If you've read the preceding chapters ("A Woman's Perspective on Infertility" and "A Man's Perspective on Infertility"), you've gained some ground in understanding your own feelings. Plus, you've got a foundation for what's going on inside the heads of most men and women. Now find out what's going on inside the head of the one you love. Talk frequently about how you are each feeling. Consider using the Mad, Sad, Glad, Scared, Hurt concept.

## Evaluating your own expectations

Everyone has preformed ideas of what they think their own family will look like. Women are more likely to come into marriage with prior expectations. What were yours? What were his?

When pregnancy doesn't happen as you expect it to, you face the death of a dream, sometimes more than one. You lose the dream that it'll be natural and easy to conceive a child. And when pregnancy never happens, you lose a lot more dreams, such as hearing a doctor confirm the news, "Yes, you're definitely pregnant!" You lose the dream of sharing the exciting news with your friends and family that "I'm pregnant!" You lose the dream of feeling a baby kick inside your body. You lose the dream of having children who will carry on your genetic characteristics.

These dreams can't just be swept aside or erased as if they never existed. To some extent, you have to grieve their losses. And yet you learn to redefine what it means to be a mother, a father; what it means to have a family; what it means to give a child a secure home. Your infertility journey makes you and your spouse work through the value of becoming a parent, the privilege of becoming a parent, much more deeply than someone who conceives right off the bat.

Take time with your spouse to discuss how easy you thought it would be to have children when you first got married, how you feel about adoption, your thoughts about infertility treatments, the possibility of living child-free.

As you think through these topics, some may need to be revisited in the months to come, after certain levels of fertility treatments have been unsuccessful, when money starts to wane, or when emotions wear paper-thin. Add questions of your own as you go along.

## Some things improve with age

Maybe not waistlines or wrinkle quotients, but some parts of your infertility journey will look a little lighter in retrospect.

Beth and Brian will be laughing for a long time at the extraordinary efforts they were prepared to go through in order to have their first child. As a minister of youth, Brian thought he might have to produce a sperm specimen at youth camp. Ministers of youth are subject to a lot of out-of-the-ordinary activities at camp, but not many have to do *that* at camp. Since the whole church knew Beth and Brian were trying to get pregnant, there was no way to keep their efforts secret. Thankfully, Beth's ovulation didn't require Brian's contribution during youth camp; but he was prepared, just in case.

Beth and Brian have found the humor in spite of the pain. One time after Beth had an insemination and was lying still on the table, Brian was there beside her and he leaned over to ask, "So, was it good for you?" Another time, after Beth became pregnant, she and Brian were out in public when they saw their fertility specialist, a woman. Brian called out, "Look! There's the lady who got my wife pregnant!"

A new perspective is one of the benefits of growing through difficulties. Some of the unusual hoops you make yourself jump through will take on a more comical light in years to come. Certainly not *all*, but a few will. Keeping track of those events in your journal will give you a plenty of fodder for your own rendition of "Then there was the time that we . . . "

You married your best friend. Remember that. Infertility puts the squeeze on your friendship. Remember that, too. God wants your marriage to do more than just survive; He wants it to thrive. After walking hand in hand through the rocky terrain of the Valley of Infertility, you can enter the next phase of your life with a marriage that will flourish because you've built stronger ties to each other through the tests and trials.

## Cara and Micah

# A marriage that didn't survive

Married in their early thirties, Cara had a plan: buy a house the first year, get furniture the second year, have a baby the third year. The first two years went just as she'd planned, so Cara went off the pill, ready to move on to phase three. But a baby didn't come in year three ... or four. Living in a city with access to fertility clinics, the couple had a place to start. Plus, they both had good jobs in real estate, so finances weren't an issue. They began with the introductory measures and moved their way up the ladder of complexity.

At first they relied on each other and their mutual commitment to God. They prayed about it every night. They read books on infertility and discussed them with each other over dinner. They really seemed to be a team.

But month after month passed with no positive results. Micah noticed Cara began showing no middle ground—she was either angry and confrontive or withdrawn and silent. He tried to find ways to open up conversations. Sometimes she wanted to spill; sometimes she was locked up tight. More and more, she wanted to be left alone to explore the Internet for groundbreaking fertility options.

"I'm desperate," she pleaded. "I've got to find something somewhere to work for us, even if I have to go to another clinic in another city."

Her increasing silence made life tense beyond belief. Micah never knew what kind of mood he'd find her in. But one day she was happier than he'd seen her in a long time. She'd found a test group she wanted to try to get in, and she'd made a preliminary appointment for the end of the week to talk with staff and see if she qualified for the parameters of the study. The clinic was in a large city about two hundred miles away. Cara decided to drive up the night before the appointment, spend the night with Meg, one of her friends from college, then make the 10:00 A.M. appointment and return home that afternoon.

Micah asked if he needed to be in on the consultation, too, but

Cara said they only needed to talk to her at first. A few days later, with medical records in hand and a light bag packed, she drove away, happy and excited about the possibilities. She planned to leave from work right after lunch. That evening, she called Micah from her cell phone to tell him she was about 10 minutes from Meg's house, so she'd made the trip without problems.

The next morning, Micah thought it'd be a nice touch to call and tell Cara he'd be praying for her during the appointment, so he dialed her cell phone. No answer. Maybe the batteries died, he thought. He called Meg's home phone, but she was caught off guard. She hadn't heard from Cara since her last Christmas newsletter. Micah kept trying the cell phone all morning as he looked through the papers on the desk, trying to find something to tell him which clinic she was going to, but nothing turned up. Micah later said it was the longest day of his life.

When Cara returned home that afternoon, her bubbly demeanor didn't last long. As Micah peppered her with questions, her alibi sunk. Her anger flared and she lashed out at Micah, screaming and accusing him of not loving her and not caring about having a baby. As she railed on, he began to put together a story he couldn't believe he was hearing. Cara had met someone online and had been emailing him for three months. The overnight trip was their first rendezvous. Micah was stunned. Cara left him the next day, and Micah learned later that she had quit her job and moved in with Darrel. She filed for divorce, unwilling to even discuss reconciliation. But she made sure she got the furniture.

In the months that followed, Micah tried to figure out where they had gone wrong. He remembered how much time Cara had spent talking about her former college roommates—their houses, their babies, their got-it-all-together lifestyle, at least that's how Cara saw it. She'd always wanted something she didn't have. Micah also saw that somewhere along the way he and Cara had stopped communicating on the same level. He was still getting used to being married, having a larger home to care for, yard work, plus a growing real estate business. He wanted to have kids, but he hadn't felt the urgency she had felt. They never really talked about that, Micah realized.

"I did everything Cara wanted me to do, made all the appointments she set up, except for one, and tried to 'perform' on the schedule she told me was required," he said. "Our sex life was awful. I'd stayed a virgin until marriage so I could experience sex only with my wife, and within a few years we were stuck in this routine where the mechanics were all that mattered."

The one appointment he'd missed had happened on the day Micah unexpectedly closed the biggest deal of his career to date. By the time he looked at his watch after the whirlwind of activities that morning, he realized he'd missed most of the appointment. "It wasn't a test for either of us, but just a consultation with another clinic," he said. "I never meant to miss the appointment, but in the long run, I thought it was a forgivable mistake. But I guess it wasn't."

*(The names and some aspects of this story have been altered at the contributor's request.)*

# Chapter 5

# Why Do They Have Children, and We Don't?

*I never was angry or felt badly toward other couples, but it truly hurt every time I got an email from friends saying they were having kids. The hardest part for me was hearing from friends who "planned" the timing of when they had children, as if they were truly in control of family planning.* —*Sherri*

"Why can she get pregnant, and I can't?" Now that's a question that has echoed through every millennium. In the Bible, Hannah asked it. Elizabeth struggled with it. Rachel cried over it. David's first wife, Michal, likely uttered it in bitter frustration. Almost every person interviewed for this book acknowledged his or her frustration over the agonizing process of "natural selection" that seems to heap fertility on some and deny it to others.

You can go over sanity's edge trying to figure out why teenagers get pregnant so easily in the back seat of a car. You probably have to slap your hand over your mouth to keep from lecturing the pregnant 15-year-old who waddles down the mall, window-shopping at the upscale maternity clothes store. Your soul screams, "Lord, this is just not fair! That girl doesn't know how to raise a child. She can't support a child, can't wisely discipline a child, can't love a child unconditionally. She's just a child herself! Lord, what were You thinking when You let her get pregnant and not me?"

What you're feeling is a combination of emotions—anger, confusion, grief, envy—customize the list as you need to. And it's understandable. Becoming a parent is vitally important to you, and now it has happened to someone else—someone who didn't have to work nearly as hard at it as you have.

As a Christian, you consider the role of parenthood to be as sacred as the marriage vows you pledged. You see how nurturing children is part of God's incredible plan, not only for the continuance of humanity but also so that children will have a part in God's kingdom work on earth. Those who are raised by godly parents have the best chance of becoming faithful, effective participants in God's ongoing mission. Parenthood, then, is one of *your* faith missions in life. And when you see how flippantly some people treat parenthood, it makes your blood boil.

Then there are people a lot like you who get pregnant and don't think twice about it. You can't get mad at them for getting pregnant. (Well, you can, but you feel rotten about it later!) How do you handle those feelings?

*Most couples we knew seemed indifferent to our position, and at times it seemed that they went to great lengths to talk about their pregnancies and babies in our presence. While we knew this was not the case, their insensitivity caused problems at the time. You find yourself avoiding situations where there will be a lot of unstructured time for talking. You know that with a group of young married couples, most of whom are either pregnant or trying to be, the subject will eventually involve who's pregnant, who's trying, when the babies are due, or how uncomfortable it is to be pregnant.*

*—Angela and Jim*

Now that you're having trouble conceiving, you see pregnant women everywhere. Welcome to the club. We've all been there.

*Pregnant women soon began to surround me everywhere I went— the mall, at work, at church. My Sunday school class spent the first 15 minutes talking about everyone in the community who was having a baby. I was in "a mood" every Sunday because I had to go to church and face my friends in Sunday school. I hated malls because baby strollers and pregnant women always seemed to bump into me.*
*—Rhonda*

*It felt like someone swung a baseball bat at me every time I learned someone else was pregnant. It hurt so much that I couldn't look at*

*or even hold other people's babies. I felt I would never have the joy of*
*holding my own. It was just too painful for me.* —Ann

*My sister-in-law would sneeze and she'd become pregnant; and no*
*matter what I did, it wasn't working for us. I hated her. If anyone*
*around me was pregnant, I was jealous. I would cross the street to*
*avoid having to get too close to a pregnant woman.* —Jane

*I tried to avoid encounters with pregnant women at all costs. I*
*stopped going to baby showers and the mall. Going to the ob/gyn's*
*office for an appointment would bring me to tears as I sat in a wait-*
*ing room full of pregnant women and their spouses.* —Linda

Lori volunteered at a crisis pregnancy counseling center
and talked with a lot of pregnant young women. She was in
the middle of infertility treatments when she became pregnant, but she lost the baby at eight weeks. Her first day back
at the counseling center, she sat face-to-face with a client who
was eight weeks pregnant and wanted an abortion. Enraged,
Lori screamed at the woman, venting her anger over the
injustice of what she had lost and what this young woman
wanted to cast aside. It wasn't fair. It never is.

### Fertile family, infertile me
You can really get your fur up when you see pregnant women
who don't value their pregnancy. But anger, even jealousy, can
overflow to couples with children, even though they have as
much right to a child as you do and who will cherish the children God gives them. Especially disturbing is when you find
yourself envying your own family members who have no
trouble conceiving.

These are the people you love the most—your own brothers
and sisters, your cousins, your aunts and uncles, your nieces
and nephews. But they are busy with children of their own—
and you with none. Certainly you love their children and in
some moments of vicarious parenthood, you may feel you
live out a little of your own parenting through them. But still,
Lord, what's the deal? Why do they conceive, and you don't?
They get pregnant at the drop of a hat, and you can't get
pregnant when you dump out your entire savings account!

My brother and his wife are the antithesis to my husband's and my infertility problems. With each of their children, Amy conceived soon after she stopped using the pill. Their first two pregnancies effortlessly progressed while we were going to great lengths to achieve our first pregnancy.

Your family members are probably cognizant of your struggles and compassionate about your ordeal. (If they just don't get it, show them this book.) But even the most compassionate people cannot truly understand a trial unless they've walked through it themselves. If they haven't experienced the depths of infertility, their ability to relate and empathize will be limited. Be grateful for any kindness shown to you, and assure the giver of your appreciation.

✷ We who battle infertility have a responsibility too. We need to control ourselves and make sure we don't get too hung up on our need to have constant sympathy poured on our inflamed wounds or to have conversations edited so that they don't mention topics that remind us of our loss. Every comment cannot be monitored for how it will affect the aching hearts of an infertile couple. Even the kindest empathizers have no idea how many subjects poke painfully at our raw hearts. Just about every subject in daily life connects in some way to children or family. Thus, everything reminds us of our loss. ✷

People who expect and demand sympathy from others can be pretty uncomfortable to be around. They are a bottomless pit of neediness, turning normal conversations into an opportunity to reiterate their woes. Receive empathy, sympathy, and kindness, but don't demand it. It's not easy to require that kind of behavior of yourself; but with grit and determination you can do it. I'm not implying you should never share your pain—you definitely should. But how and when are the keys.

### When congratulations are in order

Remember this one? "Rejoice with those who rejoice; mourn with those who mourn. Live in harmony with one another" (Rom. 12:15–16).

I nearly made a mess of things when Ted and Amy announced they were expecting their second child. A large crowd was at my parents' home, celebrating my youngest brother's high school graduation. It was a natural time for Ted and Amy to make the announcement in the presence of so many loved ones. Their two-year-old firstborn, Alexander, was moving around the group, grinning at a great-aunt, giving a high five to Grandpa, just generally being adorable. At his parents' instruction, Alexander carried a card to Grandma, my mother. The picture on the card showed two children walking hand in hand. Inside was written, "Grandma, I'm going to be a big brother. Love, Alexander."

Grandma's eyes danced with delight. Grandpa grinned ear-to-ear. Aunts, uncles, and everyone celebrated the news. But Edward and I sat on the outskirts of the circle, absolutely speechless. I somehow managed to dredge up a smile from some recess of my soul. The event is etched in my mind as one of those time-stood-still occasions. Everything shifted into slow motion as my brain tried to comprehend the implications—Ted and Amy were going to have a second child; and here we were, going on our ninth year of marriage with no children in sight.

As soon as possible, I found a discreet opportunity to slip to a back bedroom and be alone for a while. I needed some time alone to process what I'd heard. Not long after, Edward came back to the room, too. We pulled ourselves together before we went back to the family room. To my knowledge, no one perceived the heartbreaking emotions that were tumbling around inside. Edward later wrote:

*My pain was brought to the forefront again: I was not a father yet. I couldn't be fully happy for them, and I felt guilty that I couldn't. Then there was the pressure, whether real or imagined, from other family members that Cindy and I had never made this type of announcement. I hurt for Cindy because she was caught off guard. My emotions rolled over me like a wave that day. I was able to work through them in time; but in that instant, it was almost too much to handle.*

Later that afternoon, I crossed paths in a hallway as little Alexander innocently pushed around his "bubbuh maw-mow" (bubble lawn mower). He looked up at me with his clear blue eyes, and I could only look back at him in stony silence. For a split second, I perceived his surprise. This was not how Aunt Cindy usually acted! I reprimanded myself immediately. Alexander was the apple of my eye! My cubicle at work was lined with snapshots of Alexander, so much so that someone once asked me if the child in the pictures was *my son*. But now, with the announcement of his expected sibling, I was so distraught that I almost considered Alexander as someone to blame for my sadness. My conflicting emotions snapped me back to reality. I kneeled and gave Alexander a hug.

In looking back at that afternoon, I thank God that He allowed me to keep my mouth shut and not make a scene during Ted and Amy's announcement. Edward and I were terribly disappointed—not that they were pregnant, but that we were not. And it's important that we acknowledged our sorrow. Several days later we discussed our feelings with Ted and Amy, and they shared with us how unsure they'd been about how to handle the situation.

### Handle yourself with grace
"Rejoice with those who rejoice." But how do you rejoice when your heart feels like a truck rolled over it, and your throat is choking back the sobs?

For starters, when family members announce that they're expecting a baby, remember that the advent of a child is a blessing, even if that child is not yours. Even if it is *your turn* to be making the announcement. Even though it's not fair.

Give your very best effort and offer a hug to the expectant couple, even if it must be a wordless hug. If you can bring forth a word of genuine congratulations, then go for it. Keep in mind that you can always cry later, after the family gathering has dispersed. Don't let someone else's joyful announcement be overshadowed by your pain, by your flying out of the room to bury your head in a pillow and cry bitterly. Later on you'll be glad you didn't make a scene. That's a promise.

You cannot rewind and redo moments like that, as if you were rewinding and rerecording a videotape. Hold yourself together until you've retreated to a safe place to vent your disappointment. If you can clear away the confusion and anger, you might find that you're venting the grief that *you* are battling infertility, not that *they* are expecting a baby.

It may help to remember times in your life when you've been the one with the happy news and someone else had to stand by, quietly longing to experience your joy. When you announced your engagement, was a single friend wishing she could find Mr. Right? When you nailed that college scholarship, did someone who congratulated you wish he could find the resources to help him finish his education? When you found the new job that matched your skills so perfectly, did a coworker wish she could be so lucky? You haven't always been the one on the outside looking in.

### Where's the justice?

Stewing over who gets pregnant and who can't will wreak havoc on your soul. But before you belittle yourself for having these feelings, consider "from whence you've come."

Especially in the US, we think justice is an inalienable right. In some cases it is. But freedom from injustice cannot be guaranteed in all aspects of our lives. Infertility is one of those aspects. No man, woman, or fertility clinic can guarantee that only the deserving will become pregnant when they want to.

The immortal God—who *could* control the outcomes if He chose to—chooses not to prevent conception in the millions of women who have little regard for the miracle that grows within them. But do we blame God for being unjust?

Job, the most afflicted person in the Old Testament, was never faced with the struggle of infertility, but he was leveled with a lousy series of personal losses—the deaths of his children, the natural destruction of all his property and livestock, and the loss of his own health.

Job says, "'I am innocent but God denies me justice. . . . Far be it from God to do evil, from the Almighty to do wrong. . . . It is unthinkable that God would do wrong, that the Almighty would pervert justice. Who appointed him over the earth? Who put him in charge of the whole world? If it were his intention and he withdrew his spirit and breath, all mankind would perish together and man would return to the dust. . . . [God] shows no partiality to princes, and does not favor the rich over the poor, for they are all the work of his hands" (Job 34:5, 10, 12–15, 19).

We think of Job as the humble, spiritually immovable man who endured more heartache that any known human. In parts of the above passage, I wonder if Job was being cynical, in other parts angry and frustrated. Too often we read Job's words and give him a saintly voice that utters only calm words of endurance and humility. We have to remember that the guy was just as human as we are, and the losses he incurred broke his heart. Job must have wondered at least once or twice why God wasn't cutting him a little slack, even if he didn't state it in so many words.

The simple, very painful truth is that God shows no partiality to those who *deserve* to conceive. He doesn't ensure that every Christian couple will conceive a child. On the other hand, He doesn't abruptly halt the meeting of a sperm and an egg simply because the participants aren't deserving or aren't prepared to be parents. He doesn't flip the switch on a teenaged girl's rampant fertility just because she loses her virginity in the heat of immature passion.

God has a track record of not intervening at times we think He ought to. But who are we to understand the mind of the eternal, all-knowing God? Historically, He has let men and women choose their paths. And if a fertile man and a fertile woman choose to have sex, chances are great they will eventually conceive, even though sexual selfishness may be the only motivation in their relationship. God lets them choose their course. As a loving heavenly Father, He waits for His children to see the error of their selfish choices and come to Him for help, direction, and forgiveness. But never, absolutely never, does He force righteousness on anyone.

As much as our human nature wants to, we must hold our tongues before we lash out and condemn the woman who conceives in sin, the woman who conceives and then complains, or the woman who conceives easily and takes it for granted. Though some of them don't act the part, they are all creations of a loving God.

And they need to be reminded of that. They need to be nudged to understand that the gift of life that grows within them is a miraculous creation of a loving God, just as they are. They need someone to help them remove the shackles of a culture that has devalued life and undermined the esteemed role of parents. They need a gentle-spirited friend who will help them see their own value in God's eyes, so they can begin to accept the responsibility of loving and nurturing the priceless treasure that has been entrusted to them.

## Justice—the big picture

To help you settle the horrible pain in your heart, we need to get to the bottom of this need for justice. And to do that, we need to think about justice outside of its implications to infertility. We need to think bigger than that.

Justice is something doled out by a judge. And in the eternal perspective, God is the ultimate Judge.

The Bible assures us that a day will come when everyone will be judged, when all mankind will stand before the God of justice and truth . . . and love. At that time, you will look into the face of the heavenly Judge, and you will know your sinful state like you've never known it before. Standing before a perfectly holy God who has never embodied sin, you will know what it's like to feel the need for being made pure in His holy presence.

In that moment you will realize the irony—the Judge has already paid the penalty for your crimes. The Judge sent His beloved Son so that you will not be held to the letter of the law. Though the Judge has every right to throw the book at you for your waywardness (however mild it may seem when compared to other people), the Judge takes note that you, in your earthly life, realized the need for a Savior to erase your sinfulness. You are excused from the import of this heavenly judgment scene. You are pardoned from the weight of justice that could have fallen on your soul.

Justice is God's to dispense, not ours. One day Christians will be pardoned for their sins because "God so loved the world that he gave his one and only Son" (John 3:16). One day we will benefit from the love of God, Who chose not to exercise justice in its strictest sense. In that light, why are we so intent on demanding fairness be meted out as to who gets pregnant and who doesn't? This God has already proven His love to us through Jesus Christ. He can be trusted to prove His love again by granting the deepest desires of our hearts—to love a child.

Will you trust the all-knowing Judge to work in your life as He sees fit? Will you let your loving Father guide you to infertility options and parental opportunities that are in His plan for you? Will you submit to His wisdom in weaving together a tapestry in your life that will be beautiful and exquisite, even though it may not be the design you originally planned?

There are no quick fixes for the whys that infertility brings. Finding a way to personally resolve the question "Why do they have children and we don't?" will be a little different for each of us, but there's a common end result that's possible for every believer. "For a little while you may have had to suffer grief in all kinds of trials. These have come so that your faith—of greater worth than gold, which perishes even though refined by fire—may be proved genuine and may result in praise, glory and honor when Jesus Christ is revealed" (1 Peter 1:6–7).

And for those of you who have been blessed with the capacity to bear children, here are some tips for how to reach out in compassion for those of us who haven't:

## How to tell an infertile couple you're expecting:

*Don't let us hear of your pregnancy through the grapevine just because you don't quite know how to tell us face-to-face.* It's far more painful for us to hear it from someone else. We will appreciate the fact that you trust us with your news and that you love us enough to make sure we're not caught off guard during the announcement.

*If you plan to make the announcement in a group setting, tell us prior to the event.*
Give us a day or so before the event to process the information and pull ourselves together emotionally. We really want to be supportive of you, but our emotions are a little unpredictable.

*Tell us privately, not in a restaurant or a hallway at church.*
Share your news somewhere out of the public eye, where we can ask you questions, and maybe even get a little teary-eyed without being self-conscious.

# An uncommon bond of motherhood

When Bobbi McCaughey birthed septuplets in November 1997, the world took notice. Amazingly, the couple, their doctors, and their church kept the news to themselves until the end of Bobbi's pregnancy. But once the impending births were announced, the media blitz exploded and you couldn't get away from the story on any channel (except perhaps ESPN). Ken and Bobbi boldly testified to reporters that, as Christians, they could not justify terminating the lives of any of the babies (selective reduction), so they determined early on to accept the responsibility of a large multiple birth.

When I saw the televised images of seven babies cradled in every inch of space in both parents' arms, my inner voice cried, "But, Lord, I'm just asking for *one!*" I didn't begrudge them their seven newborns, but why couldn't God give me just one little baby? We'd already endured years of infertility and one failed adoption. The struggle flared again over life's unjust and unfair outcomes.

Within months of the septuplets' births, God opened my eyes to the underside of the tapestry He had been weaving beyond my understanding. While I was crying to Him about the unfairness of Bobbi birthing her seven on November 19, the mother of our child had already given birth on November 5, though we wouldn't learn about Ryan's existence until January 1998. Bobbi and Ken's babies were tiny indeed, yet we later compared birth weights and realized our Ryan weighed less than any of the septuplets. Their seven and our one stayed in neonatal intensive care units on opposite sides of the country for about the same amount of time. Like Ryan, some of their children came home on supplemental oxygen. The McCaugheys juggled oxygen, heart monitors, and more—and so did we. As the McCaugheys face raising several children who have special needs as a result of their unusual birth, we have accepted the responsibility of raising our premature son who also has special needs.

In the fall of 1997, while I was bemoaning what I didn't have in common with Bobbi McCaughey, God was putting together the details of an adoption He was about to hand to us. In retrospect, I think I have quite a bit in common with Bobbi now.

In the midst of confusing darkness, we must remind ourselves that we never know where and how God is at work, weaving together people and events. In time He will show us the underside of His incredible tapestry.

# Chapter 6

# Grief—Wandering through the Maze

*The teenaged girl who chose us to be her child's parents confessed during one of our meetings that earlier in her pregnancy she had hit her stomach, hoping to cause a miscarriage. We continued working with her until the baby was born. But right before she was to place him in our arms, she changed her mind and decided to keep him. Perhaps more than our own pain of losing a child, we grieve for the plight of this baby, who is now living with a mother who abused him before he was even born.*
*—Patty*

The grief you experience during your infertility journey is like a maze of tall hedges. As you wander your way down its narrow path, you can't see which direction leads to the way out of your pain. All you can do is make a choice here and there and continue trudging along.

Every person's experience with grief is unique because every person and every situation is different. Two women in infertility treatments may both experience miscarriages, but their grief journeys will not be identical. They have different backgrounds, expectations, temperaments, and outlooks. We must never say, "I know exactly how you feel" when someone has experienced loss. We cannot know exactly how he or she feels. A better response would be: "I remember what it felt like when I (had a miscarriage, learned I was infertile, etc.). I'm so sorry you've experienced this loss."

Though grief is *expressed* with individuality, some common themes exist in each grief experience: shock, denial, anger, depression, bargaining, and acceptance. The grief process is a journey where we move in and out, back and forth, across and over these phases as we work our way toward a new emotional balance. Each phase is not characterized by a clear beginning and ending, but rather a blending from one to another, overlapping and intertwining along the way.

The journey may have a specific beginning, such as a miscarriage or a specific test result, but the grief of infertility doesn't have a specific ending. The loss of a child, a pregnancy, or your dreams is something that you weather and survive, but it's not something you forget and leave behind. It's a part of what defines your life story.

For example, you may think you've emotionally recovered from a miscarriage, when months or years later, strong and distressing feelings can resurface, similar to when you were initially dealing with the loss. "Grief spasms," according to one author, are moments when a person is thrown back to those initial, overwhelming feelings. But if you've allowed yourself to work through your grief, then the grief spasm won't last as long or be as intense as your first experience.

So how do you work through it the first time? You need to learn how to take care of your emotional needs as they arise.

### Take care of yourself

Beth Herrian is a psychotherapist in Texas who counsels families and individuals through various kinds of crises. She herself is a veteran of crisis. Beth and her husband, Brian, battled infertility for years before they finally birthed Corban in 1997.

Brian was a minister of youth. "Everybody at church knew we were trying to get pregnant," Beth says. "We had good friends who acted as a barrier, a buffer for us, so we wouldn't have to answer the same questions forty-two times. But still, anytime someone cautiously asked 'So, how are you doing?' I knew they really wanted to know if we were pregnant yet."

With a background in counseling and psychology, you might wonder if all that education helped Beth breeze through the grief of her own infertility. Hardly. Having knowledge and understanding of grief didn't lessen the pain, she says, "although it did allow me to identify my emotions as they were occurring—'Oh, this is *anger* I'm feeling right now!' I knew that these feelings were okay, that they were a normal part of grief. But it didn't stop me from hurting or from experiencing those emotions."

But the key question, Beth believes, is, "What do I need to do to take care of myself right now?" This question is central. In working your way through infertility's grief, ask yourself what you need to do at that moment to cope with your pain. Do you need to find a quiet spot and cry out the tension that's keeping you knotted up internally? Do you need to go for a walk or jog? Do you need to spend some time soaking up peace from God's Word? Maybe you need to journal, to treat yourself to a long bubble bath, to call up a friend who's been through infertility, or to sit down with your spouse and just hold each other.

Think right now about what brings you emotional relief. Anticipate that on some days you'll need to do something to relieve your heart of its pain. Make a list ahead of time, to prepare for those days. Remember the list, refer to it, and give yourself permission to take care of your needs.

### Grief and loss

"Grief comes from loss. You can grieve job loss, loss of a position, relocation, loss of a loved one," Beth says. "But with infertility, you've lost not only the child you may have carried, but the dream of the child you want to carry, the child you can't conceive."

Women, particularly, have many dreams associated with motherhood: the dream of telling people you're pregnant (especially your husband), the dream of feeling a baby kick for the first time, the dream of having a seconds-old newborn laid on your chest. A million dreams. A million ways to feel loss.

"With infertility, the hardest thing is that you feel loss every month," Beth says. The emotional roller coaster takes you from the hopeful highs to the disheartening lows in a four-week time frame. Depending on the person, the intensity of infertility's grief may or may not outrank the intensity of other kinds of grief. But, Beth says, we must remember: "Grief is grief, and loss is loss. They all hurt."

And no matter what the grief is, we go through it one day at a time. We cope with it one day at time. And we survive it one day at a time. Don't bite off any more than one day. And some days, you need to nibble on even less—just try to survive an hour, a moment—and that's okay. These are unbelievably hard experiences you're dealing with. Don't let anyone tell you otherwise.

### God can be trusted with your unknown reality

Grief and grieving have taken on negative connotations in our language because their very mention brings up dark, dismal images of encounters with death or tragedy. But the experience of grieving is actually a path toward healing, of coming to terms with the loss in your life. It's not just *important* for you to grieve your loss; it's vitally *necessary* to do so.

Grieving is the active effort on your part to process the loss you've experienced—active in that you let yourself experience the pain and sadness, you come face-to-face with the reality of what is lost (or is being lost every month), and you honestly assess your feelings at a hundred points along the way.

The opposite of this would be choosing to deny the reality of what has been lost, of not facing the unknown reality that your loss has pushed you into. Many people bail out of their grief process by finding escape routes. Some deny their grief by pushing it down every time it surfaces.

As Christians, we can trust that no matter how painful and devastating our grief, we need not fear the unknown reality brought about by our loss. To feel fear along the way is natural, but to linger in a state of fear is evidence that we need to draw from the reservoirs of peace offered by our all-knowing God. Although we are frustrated, devastated, and angered by the pain that God has allowed to come into our lives, we can walk—or sometimes crawl—through the grief process, knowing that our ever-faithful Lord is walking beside us even when we don't sense His problem-solving intervention. He *is* there with us, and He *can* be trusted to usher us into the future.

### Grief protracted, expanded, and elongated

Infertility is a war against the circumstances and conditions that keep you from bringing forth *life*; and, ironically, most people characterize infertility's grief as a series of *deaths*—the death of your dreams, your hopes, your desires. Your loss is not a onetime event, like the death of an elderly relative, but a series of experiences over a period in your life. Grieving through your infertile years means coming to terms with any number of losses along the way—month after month of not getting pregnant, miscarriages, failed inseminations, failed in vitros, failed adoptions, and more. The events often tumble on top of each other so you don't have the chance to grieve one loss before the next one hits.

Infertility requires us to grieve on several levels at once. While you're coming to terms with the loss of your expectations (that pregnancy could happen normally), you may enter the grief related to a miscarriage. It's compounded by the month-after-month drain on your emotional bank as infertility treatments wear on and on.

So how do we get a handle on this kind of grief? Thomas Attig, a professor at Bowling Green State University in Kentucky who teaches courses on grief issues, believes we must look at grief as something we *do*:

*On all accounts, our grieving is thought of as something that we do. We do not remain passive but rather actively engage the challenges presented by our longing for, and need to let go of, those we care about. We struggle to find means of overcoming, gaining control of, or constructively expressing and directing our emotions. We work our way through crises in self-identity and disruptions in our usual behavior patterns and develop alternatives. We address and seek to overcome strains in relationships and to build new ones. And we seek ways to make sense of our new reality and to find meaning in life without the deceased.*

When we consider that grief is not just a state that we're *in*, but see it also as something we must *do*, then we can consider that how we feel and act during our grief is actually constructive behavior that moves us toward healing. The pain, then, has a purpose.

The various phases of grief can come in any order, can resurface again and again, and can pass slowly or quickly. The next section of this chapter explains more about these phases and what you'll feel or experience. My hope is that by understanding the phases, you'll feel more in control of your journey. For example, if you can deduce that your sudden outburst of impatience over something trivial was really caused by your anger that you've just started your period again, then you've helped to restore some order in your life. Reestablishing some measure of order, predictability, or routine helps us to move forward out of the confusion of grief.

### Feelings of shock and denial

It's not unusual to go through a period of numbness when you first discover your infertility. For some of us, it's like a slow dawning as we realize that pregnancy is not happening as quickly as it should. For others, it's the shock and disbelief that comes from the result of one test that shows an inadequacy. Surely this can't be happening to *you*! We may deny this new reality by trying to prove it wrong: "We'll work really hard in the next few months and we'll get pregnant, you just wait and see."

"So much about denial is fear," Beth says. "We deny it because we're afraid of what it can mean. When you start looking at your fear, you see you're afraid you'll never have children, afraid you've lost control over your future. Deal with denial by dealing with the fear. Fear immobilizes. Face the fear and look at what's behind it. Then you can make plans and start moving."

### Ways to cope:

"Do some reading on infertility, either on the Internet or at the library," Beth suggests. "You think you're the only one feeling this way, so you need to find out that it's happened to other women like you—intelligent, upwardly mobile women. During this phase you probably don't want to have much to do with people labeled *infertile*, so you may not feel up to going to a support group meeting. But you can read and learn while still keeping your distance."

At this stage of the game, Beth suggests that you choose carefully the people you tell about your infertility. "Don't subject yourself to the advice you'll encounter from everyone," she says. "You need someone who will just listen to you, not try to give you all the answers."

Beth is an advocate of journaling. "Keeping a journal brings out the feelings you didn't even know were there." If you've never journaled, you really need to give it a try. Writing down your feelings is a surprisingly freeing process. You don't have to be eloquent or even careful. Just write whatever you feel. Write out your prayers to God. Write anything.

Now, if you're one of those who is repulsed at the thought of buying a cute little cloth-covered journal, you still have no excuse. You can journal on anything, anywhere—a tiny spiral notebook stuffed in your purse to jot down quick feelings or thoughts; the back of the church bulletin, where you write down how you feel as you watch the baby dedication; the napkin you scribble on at the restaurant when a helpful analogy comes to mind; the back of the grocery list. No excuses. Just journal.

### How to handle your feelings of anger

Your anger may be directed in several ways: at yourself, at others, at God. First of all, *own* your anger. Admit that you're angry. Anger that's not dealt with, that gets turned inward, can turn into depression.

"When I have depressed people in my office, I ask, 'What are you angry about?' " Beth says. "A lot of times they'll say, 'I'm not angry; I'm depressed!' But when I press on, I find anger that's never been dealt with. Behind anger you find emotions that have never been addressed."

Beth explains the pyramid that leads to depression. The bottom layer is the basic emotions that result from a problem or incident. Infertility brings fear, frustration, and pain. The next layer in the pyramid is the anger that results from those feelings. And if those feelings are never properly addressed, the pinnacle of the pyramid will eventually form and be manifested as depression.

You may be angry at yourself because your body has let you down in this all-important role of reproduction. You're frustrated that your life has clipped along at a nice, predictable pace, but now your plans have fallen apart. You're afraid you've lost control of your future and your dreams.

Your anger may be aimed at your husband, who doesn't understand why you're so consumed by your quest for motherhood. Or maybe he's angry at you because he doesn't share your timetable on how to approach infertility.

You may be angry at your doctors. *Why can't they make me get pregnant? Why am I emptying my bank account and they're still not able to make this work right?* Fertility specialists are like soldiers on the front line of battle. They stand a good chance of getting shot at.

Finally, your anger is likely to be aimed at God: *Why aren't You letting me get pregnant? Why is everyone pregnant but me?*

"Being angry with God is okay," Beth says. "His shoulders are big enough to handle it. Anger is not a sin, but what we do with anger can become sin." Anger with God comes from our wanting to know why this is happening to us. We want answers and we're not getting them."

## Ways to cope:
Find safe ways to vent your anger. Stuffing it, ignoring it, and hoping it will go away does absolutely no good. It *will* erupt sooner or later, and later will be much worse than sooner because the pain will have festered and infected your soul in the meantime.

"Run, exercise, write, draw, even scream at God if you want to," Beth suggests. "He'd rather you talk to Him in anger than not talk to Him at all." (See chapter 12, "Spiritual Implications of Infertility," for more on handling your anger toward God.)

## The temptation to bargain
When someone in grief tries to find ways to negotiate the situation into a more positive resolution, that's bargaining. We try to bargain with God, with ourselves, and with others.

Bargaining with God might be displayed as a woman who tries to be a spiritual superwoman as a way to earn God's favor for answered prayer. *If I start having a quiet time, if we start going to church on Sunday night, if I volunteer more at church. . . .* The problem is that bargaining with God becomes a works-based mentality: "If I do something for God, then He will be more inclined to answer my prayers for parenthood." It's like buying God's favor with our actions. But it doesn't work that way.

If your underlying reason for doing increased spiritual gymnastics is to evoke a predictable response from God (i.e., pregnancy) then your reasons are self-serving. And since God has His own timetable and master plan, He's going to answer your prayers when it suits Him. If you make changes in your spiritual life for the wrong reasons, and then see that God isn't acquiescing to your not-so-subtle demands, you'll only frustrate yourself and end up more angry at God.

We bargain with ourselves when we throw our hopes into one arena and begin working feverishly to eliminate every possible reason we're not getting pregnant. A woman might go on a massive health food kick, eliminating caffeine, chocolate, coffee, or trying natural products that claim to boost fertility. Or maybe she starts exercising fanatically to get that extra weight off, just in case that's affecting her fertility. If she suspects her job is the culprit, causing stress that might be limiting her fertility, she may take a leave of absence or resign.

Couples who have encountered many failures and decreasing options may bargain against fate by throwing themselves into an all-out search for a fertility clinic with better statistical results, newer techniques, or doctors who are willing to try again and again.

**Ways to cope:**
It's always a good idea to get yourself right with God. If you need to straighten out, firm up, or reestablish your walk with Him, go for it. But do it for the right reasons, not to persuade God to do something for you. Spend some time reading about God's character—His awesome nature, His holiness, His unending love for you. Contemplate just who He is. (This might help deter you from thinking you can manipulate Him!) Ask yourself if your need to bargain with God has at its core a basic lack of trust in the plan He has for your life. Fearing what He has in store can send you into a tailspin of self-directed activity that is intent on accomplishing *your* goals at any and all costs.

**Identify feelings of acceptance**
Most couples who have not conquered infertility will eventually work their way toward feelings of acceptance in regard to their infertility. Acceptance doesn't mean they *like* this new reality, but they can consider the change with more emotional balance than before.

Perhaps they've adopted, chosen to foster a child, or come to terms with living without children. Acceptance doesn't mean they like being classified as infertile, but it indicates that they have adjusted (or are in the process of adjusting) to a different reality for life. For example, you can acknowledge the fact that you will likely never bear children, become pregnant, or pass along your genetic code to your offspring.

"It's important to realize that you're going to come in and out of feelings of acceptance," Beth says. "You're going to be more okay with it some days than others. But overall, you'll reach a level where you're more content than discontent. Your lows aren't as low or as long as they were before."

## Make the pain go away

When my father passed away, we had known about his cancer for only twenty-nine days. There was no possible way we had accepted the coming end of his life. Looking back, I can see that we were still bargaining with God and man—desperately bargaining. Doctors tried procedures until they could do nothing more, so we began searching for answers on our own, investigating alternative approaches to curing cancer, exploring ways to kill the cells that were robbing us of our future with Dad. We brought him home from the hospital, and he died in his sleep before the sun rose the next day. We were shocked. We were angry. We were numb.

Sitting in a Christian counselor's office the week after Dad's funeral, my mother, youngest brother, and I asked the counselor how to get through this horror, to get past the awful way we were feeling.

"You want to *stop* feeling this way?" he asked.

I remember wanting to say, with all the inflection of a teenager with an attitude, "Well *duh*, yes! Of course we want the pain to stop! What do you think we're here for?"

He rather bluntly explained to us that to remove the pain would stifle the grief process. Though the pain felt bad, it was a part of the healing that would come. We talked for almost two hours to him and left without feeling significantly better. But about a year later, I saw the wisdom in what he said. We had wanted to just escape the pain. We knew we couldn't bring Dad back, but we hoped the counselor would hold some biblical or psychological insight that would make us feel less pain.

The only way to feel better after experiencing loss is to allow yourself to feel horrible for a while. The grief process is one that must be walked through fully. Too many people squelch their pain because they think it's going to overwhelm and destroy them. Too many people stop the grief process because they fear it will destroy their faith, rather than rest in the truth that their faith will survive. Too many people just don't trust themselves to survive grief.

There's no formula for determining how long grief will last for each person, but Beth has observed that six to twelve months is a fairly average length of time for most people who have lost someone close to them. "You also have to take into account whether it was a timely death or an untimely one," she says, referring to whether the death (or loss) was expected or if it came as a complete surprise.

## Surviving miscarriage or neonatal death

The pain of losing an unborn or newborn child is quite real. Many people don't grasp that completely. Couples encountering stillbirth (technically, week 20 to birth) have unique, difficult decisions to make that miscarriage sufferers do not. These couples must determine if they will see the baby and if they will have a funeral or even a simple prayertime to commemorate their child's existence. The key: whatever is most comforting for the parents is what should be done.

Parents can choose to see their deceased infant after birth, even if medical staff recommends against it (due to physical abnormalities, etc.). Seeing their child's face and holding him in their arms can help immensely with closure, giving identity to this little one they were awaiting. Taking a picture of each parent holding the baby may bring some parents great comfort in the years to come.

Naming the baby attributes personhood to him. Finding ways to remember his life helps parents move forward. One woman finally found closure to her newborn's death by naming him—30 years after he died. My sister-in-law lost twin girls, but she and her husband named them Stephanie and Chelsea. Each girl has an angel ornament on the Christmas tree. Other parents find comfort in writing an occasional letter to the child they have lost, expressing their love for him.

## Coping with lost embryos

Technology has increased our infertility options, but with it comes a wave of ethical implications—and grief possibilities. A generation ago, infertile couples tried inseminations, but never knew if fertilization occurred unless pregnancy resulted. Now with IVF, ICSI, and ZIFT procedures, couples know if eggs are fertilized, if embryos are healthy, and likewise, when they die.

Yet the grief from losing embryos is rarely discussed or acknowledged, whether they were lost naturally, in the lab, or through selective reduction (a controversial procedure which eliminates implanted embryos to improve survival rates of the remaining ones). Embryos are so "early in the game" that most people unfamiliar with infertility's struggles have a hard time recognizing the loss as a valid reason for grief. But what everyone else thinks doesn't matter. If, besides grieving a failed IVF, you need to grieve the deaths of embryos, do it. Find a meaningful way to remember those microscopic dots of life that were the combined genes of you and your spouse. Would it help to assign a gender and a name to them? Would it comfort you to imagine that they, tiny as they were, were just as precious in God's sight as any other baby? Well, it's true.

## Wading through a failed adoption

A couple pursuing adoption has likely already known the grief of infertility, maybe even miscarriage or neonatal loss. To step into the arena of adoption puts their hearts on the line for another kind of grief. Like pregnancy, an adoption can fall apart at many points along to way. Or, as Patty explained at the beginning of this chapter, a couple may have reason to grieve that the child's life is in danger from abuse or neglect.

Joy and Jeff were matched with a birth mother. When she went into labor, the couple went to the hospital and named the baby girl at birth. But they quickly realized the birth mother's family was not entirely supportive of her adoption plan. Several days later, the teenaged girl decided to keep the baby. Joy and Jeff have had two successful, problem-free adoptions.

With failed adoption, a couple encounters a different level of grief wholly unlike the grief of losing a baby in pregnancy. The child is not dead, but neither is the child with them. Prayer is a necessity to come to terms with the loss. Don't hesitate to get counseling if you're having trouble letting go.

### Navigating through grief: A lifelong journey

Thomas Attig wrote, "We will never be 'over' having lost those we have cared about, since the mysteries of life, death, and suffering remain untouched by our coping. We will have occasion to grieve our losses until we ourselves die." But there is hope, as he goes on to say, "Although we have little to no choice in bereavement, choice pervades our grieving. We again and again choose among alternative steps into our futures. We do not, and cannot, cope with the whole world at once. Reshaping our daily lives and changing course in our biographies are ongoing projects, never finally settled."

Which brings us back to the maze of hedges. Like the intricacies of infertility, the uneven path is strewn with fallen branches and loose gravel to trip you up and send you to your hands and knees, scraped and bruised. You can't get through infertility without being injured in some way. Release the hope or expectation that you can conceal your heart and avoid feeling pain or grief. You, like the rest of us, will figure out how to navigate this precarious path . . . one step at a time.

*Cathy and Larry*

# Coping with Loss

Married in their mid-twenties, Cathy and Larry had been married only nine months when their son, Lucas, was born seventeen weeks early. His due date was April 17, 1989, but tiny Lucas was born December 20, 1988.

"My doctor told me during labor that he had no chance," Cathy remembers. Neonatal technology hadn't developed enough to give Lucas a fighting chance, and he died during birth. Cathy was told she had an incompetent cervix and would always have problems carrying a child to term.

"I was stunned. No woman in my family ever had trouble carrying to term, or at least that's what I thought. Later I discovered that in years past, several relatives had lost their first child due to premature birth, but it was never discussed. If I had been warned, things could have been different for Lucas."

After losing Lucas, Cathy wanted to keep trying to have children, but Larry was afraid of losing another baby. "Burying a baby is so terribly painful," Cathy said. "It's not the 'Oh well, back to the drawing board' experience that outsiders assume it is. Why couldn't I have my baby in my arms instead of him being in a cemetery?" Cathy asked God *why* a million times.

Several years later Cathy carried to term and gave birth to Sam. When Sam was four, Larry and Cathy tried again, but she miscarried. Larry was adamant about not conceiving again. So Cathy and Larry began fostering children.

Then, when Sam was eight, Cathy was shocked to learn she was pregnant again, even though she and Larry were not trying to conceive. In order to carry baby Ian to term, Cathy had surgery, bed rest, at-home monitoring, several hospital stays, and a pump to administer anticontraction medications every three hours. But it was all worth it when Ian was born healthy and without complications.

Cathy's problem was a failure to carry to term. "It doesn't do much good to get pregnant if you can't stay that way," Cathy says. "Not many days go by when I don't think about Lucas—what he would look like, how he would get along with Sam and Ian, what he would be like as a person. I get weepy around his birthday, but usually by December 20 I'm in control again. Nobody even seems to remember he ever existed except for me and Larry."

"When most people find out I lost a baby, they say things like, 'Well, it's not like losing a real child because you never even knew him.' But that's just the point! I never got to see him smile or hear him laugh. I never even got to feel him take a breath. I realize it's hard for people to know what to do or say, but parents don't forget the babies they lost, and they don't want other people acting as if the child somehow 'didn't count.'"

How would she like people to remember Lucas? A few weeks after Lucas was born, Cathy learned that a friend had put a children's book in her church library in memory of him. "That was nice, and yes, flowers on his grave would be nice, too," Cathy said. "It's not that I want people bringing him up continually. That would be very painful. But when it's almost his birthday, I wish people could at least remember and understand why I feel that way. If on his birthday, someone would just say, 'How is it today?' or 'How old would he have been today?' it would help."

Cathy remembers a man from work who, when he found out about Lucas, said very gently and sincerely, "It would kill me to lose my four-year-old son. But how awful it would be if I had never had those four years with him to know and love him."

"Someone who can understand like that," Cathy said, "without having you explain things in detail—that person comes straight from the heart of God."

# Chapter 7

# Setting Boundaries in the Valley of Infertility

*We've drawn the line and decided not to do any more fertility treatments since we just discovered I have a disorder that could make another pregnancy a very high risk for both me and the baby. After two miscarriages and one birth, we now see that our little boy is even more of a miracle.*

*—Celeste and Mike*

When I grasped my high school diploma and flipped my tassel from one side to the other, I symbolically and literally put one role behind me forever and took on the next role in life. No longer a high school senior, I was going to be a college freshman. There was no in-between-ness, no fluctuation between being a high school student by day and a college student by night. I knew exactly where the boundary was between high school and college: the graduation ceremony.

However, the Valley of Infertility should be called the Land of Fuzzy Boundaries. I didn't just wake up one morning and realize I was no longer fertile. Infertility was a truth that dawned slowly as time passed and pregnancy remained elusive. Being infertile was a role I gradually took on, one I began to relate to in stages.

Though infertility is a condition that couples acknowledge progressively, you may wake up one morning, remember you've been trudging along in the Valley of Infertility, and realize your internal compass is all out of whack. That early morning stroke of perspective will cause you to think back to the person you used to be—emotionally stable, financially prepared, *in control*—and begin to question where you are now and, more important, *who* you are. Your rationale and logic are no longer strong anchors holding you steady in the gale-force winds of confusion. Your decision-making abilities are shattered in the complexity of emotions that run rampant. Somewhere along the way you've crossed some barriers you didn't even know were there.

That's why I'm a firm believer in setting some boundaries for yourself before you wade too deeply into the valley. If you're on the front end of your infertility experiences, you're in a prime position to assess where you want to lay down the boundaries now, before things get fuzzy and perplexing in the midst of treatments. But if you've already been in the valley for a while, you can still look over the land you've covered and determine where to set the boundaries from this point on. It's never too late to reclaim some measure of control over your actions and determine your level of participation in the infertility problem-solving process.

**Emotional** boundaries help you know what's really important to you. **Time** boundaries determine how long you'll try various stages of infertility treatments before moving to other options. **Financial** boundaries establish how much money you'll invest in the process of becoming parents.

### Emotional boundaries

The first invisible boundaries you'll cross will be the emotional ones. Even before your first diagnostic test, you've already had months, maybe years, of trying to get pregnant on your own. You studied the calendar and really tried to hit the exact day of ovulation. Maybe you tried the temperature chart approach after reading a book about it. Maybe you even adjusted your diet, lost weight, took vitamins or herbal supplements, or tried a homeopathic approach to curing infertility. But nothing worked, and you had no choice but to seek out a fertility specialist.

So by the time you walk in for your first consultation, you've already been battling the "Big-I monster" for a while. Your emotions have known highs and lows, but now your infertility journey is advancing to the next level. The more tests and procedures you require, the more infertility will burrow into your emotional armor like a fiercely stubborn mole. And one day you'll burst into tears or want to throw something across the room because you're frustrated, tired, and angry that you have to go through all this to become a parent.

To help regain some feeling of control over your emotions, you need to set some emotional boundaries. You can't "clep out" of the emotional duress the way some students clep out of academic courses. You have to wade through it all, but you can determine how much you want to put yourself through. Here are a few things you should ask yourself.

**What is really important to you: Being a parent or being a parent of a child you've birthed?** This one is a biggie, and it's going to require some serious discussion with your spouse and some serious reflection on your own part. Some women long to experience pregnancy and birth, and some discover they can live with skipping that part, opting to go right to holding a baby in their arms via adoption. Some men have a strong desire to pass along a genetic lineage, but some just want to have a little girl or boy call them "Daddy." Where are you along that continuum?

*The most helpful thing someone said to me was "Do you want to be pregnant or do you want a baby?" It really helped me to confirm the direction we were leaning toward, so that we could go ahead and listed ourselves with the adoption agency. Nine months later, we were holding Alex.*
*—Joy*

If you're hungering to experience pregnancy and childbirth, then you'll probably keep fighting for a pregnancy until it's successful or until the money runs out. On the other hand, if you can separate your feelings and focus on the lifelong responsibility and joys of parenthood (as opposed to the mere forty [plus or minus] weeks you'll carry a baby), then the quest of parenthood has more potential for success because you can find peace with nonbirth options such as adoption.

Find out what's most important to you and your spouse. Don't know how to get a conversation rolling? A starting place is to read aloud and openly discuss the chapters, "A

Woman's Perspective on Infertility" and "A Man's Perspective on Infertility." Why read them aloud? Because it gives you a chance to hear your wife read what women struggle with most, and it gives you a chance to hear your husband put into words the needs that men face most often with infertility. What do you agree with in the chapter? Which topic isn't an issue for you? The point is to open up conversational venues that lead you to discuss how you feel about birth and non-birth options for becoming parents.

*Where will you draw the line on pursuing a biological child?* In other words, how much will you put yourself through emotionally and physically before you reach your limits? How long is your fuse?

Compared to most of my infertile friends, my fuse must not be very long. We opted out of further treatments much earlier than most folks. I saw the emotional plummets they made, and I didn't want to put myself or my marriage through that. But other issues may spur you to say, "Enough."

*I prayed for a clear understanding of God's will as to how we should proceed and when we should get off the infertility merry-go-round. Fertility is an area of science that is changing daily. Just because something is medically possible doesn't mean it is right biblically or ethically. I wanted to know God's boundaries for us.* —Paula

One time I got a phone call just four days before Mother's Day, telling me that a friend had her second miscarriage. Already she and her husband were in their mid-thirties, struggling to bring even one pregnancy to fruition. Though they're still planning to work with a fertility clinic, I sense they are drawing a boundary line emotionally. They are exploring adoption agencies.

You may decide you'll do everything up to the point of in vitro fertilization (IVF). Or maybe you'll draw the line after you've tried it once. Chapter 9 gives details on the various medications and procedures, and how some of them can make you feel. After reading that chapter, you may have a better idea of where you want to establish a boundary.

## Time boundaries

Rather than draw boundaries based on emotional issues, you can set a limit on how long you'll try fertility treatments before moving on. The passage of time is one way we measure our lives. We celebrate anniversaries, birthdays, and milestones. But keeping tabs on how long you've been battling infertility is one of those dismal mile markers. Most of all, you wonder how long it will be before you reach your destination of parenthood.

*We decided our limit would be two years of treatment before we would go on to adoption. We figured that since I was already in my mid-thirties, two more years would mean my fertility rate had continued downward, and we would be trying harder with less fertility in our favor.* —Lou Ann

*When did you start trying to have a child?* In your journal (or in the margin of this book), jot down the approximate date you began letting down your guard to see if pregnancy would "just happen." When did you stop using contraceptives? Specialists generally agree that most couples can conceive within a year of having unprotected intercourse without giving any attention to ovulation timing. After giving randomly timed intercourse a chance, when did you start following the calendar more closely? Keeping track of the time you've invested thus far in the infertility journey will help you keep your perspective on future involvement.

*Begin thinking of an age or a date when you will say, "Enough."* Looking ahead a few years, what will be your enough-is-enough date? I remember thinking that if I wasn't pregnant by about 35, then I would stop whatever treatments we were in and move to adoption. Thirty-five was a mile marker for me, a personal stopping point in the future. Where (or when) do you want to place your boundary?

## Financial boundaries

Even though the word *money* has five letters, in the infertility battle it can carry all the bad vibes of a four-letter word. Money can be one of the most frustrating aspects of battling infertility because beating it can require a lot of that green paper stuff.

Many couples' quest for a biological child erases their entire savings account, then they go on to borrow money from relatives or institutions. Others plunk it all down for adoption fees. Either way, a boundary line has been crossed. How do you find balance in appropriating money for infertility measures? How do you set your financial boundaries so that you have a peace about what you spend and where you draw the line? What are your feelings about bringing a child into a financially troubled family?

As advanced as infertility technology has become, an inherent problem still exists: No one can tell you how much money you need to spend to correct your infertility problems. No one, not even your doctor. Your situation may seem identical to another couple who became pregnant after only two inseminations, but there are absolutely no guarantees that you'll get pregnant as quickly or inexpensively. Treating infertility is a lot like gambling: The enticement is always there—what will happen *the next time?* If just one more procedure will be the one to bring about a successful pregnancy, if you could know for certain it would really work, then of course it would be worth every penny. But you just can't know that. No one but God knows that.

"But isn't a child worth any cost? We'll have the rest of our lives to pay off loans, but we only have a few years before the biological clock plays out." You'll get no argument from me— a child's value is off the scale. But the question isn't about a child's worth. The question is about the cost of the *process* of getting a child. And since there's more than one process you can explore to become parents, you have to determine where to plunk down your money for the best results.

Pushing yourself into one more . . . one more . . . just one more infertility procedure is a little like the incentive that draws someone to insert just a little more money into the slot machine and give the wheels another roll. In both scenarios, the anticipation is always that the next time you might be the big winner. The unknown pulls you forward to try again and again.

## Setting boundaries on your bank account

Let's get right to the central issue: Are you bringing this financial situation to God regularly? You probably ask God daily to give you a baby, but have you sought Him regarding the money you're spending (or considering spending) on infertility treatments?

It's a stewardship issue when you get down to the nitty gritty. God has entrusted you with abilities: the ability to love and parent a child and the ability to make money to assist you in becoming a parent. The question is, does God want you to spend your very last dime (plus some borrowed ones) to embrace your parental abilities? How many dimes *does* He want you to spend?

No clear-cut answer exists. Every couple needs to determine an answer for themselves because every situation (and every bank account) differs. Rarely does anyone consider costs at the outset; and before they know it, they've immersed themselves in deeper and deeper treatments (and expenses), and now their quest for a baby is so intense, their powers of financial reasoning are mute.

Wherever you are in the process, here are a few questions to consider in setting financial boundaries that work for you.

*What is your current financial situation—outstanding debt, savings, income, expenses?* Now is the time to get your finances in order if you've never done it. Assess your income, expenses, debt, and savings. What are your spending requirements? What are your spending habits? Determine where you need to cut back to funnel more into savings. Money management books and planning helps are abundant at your local bookstore. Some excellent ones are written by and for Christians and will have a God-centered approach to money management. Whatever it takes and whomever you need to talk to, get your financial situation on paper or on your computer, and get a real-life assessment of where you stand.

*What is the status of your home, cars, etc.?* If you and your spouse are driving vehicles on the edge of extinction, consider the likelihood that someone's car will permanently croak right in the middle of your infertility expenses. Call it Murphy's

Law, bad luck, or coincidence, but don't close your eyes and hope all the problems go away until after you've birthed a child.

If your bathroom is in the middle of a major remodeling, think carefully before you decide to halt the tile job and start paying for infertility treatments. One spouse may think a half-finished bathroom is no big deal, but it could become a source of contention for the other spouse who's stressed to the max with infertility worries. In other words, do what you can to shore up the unfinished projects or problem areas.

Think about trading in the tired, old cars for one good vehicle and carpool to work. Finish up the remodeling project you're working on and don't start another one. Everyone agrees that infertility saps you of more than money—it eats away at your emotional stability with lightning speed. Don't let high-cost projects or problems be a potential disaster area for the emotional aspect of your marriage.

*How does each partner feel about spending money on infertility treatments?* Both of you need to verbalize your opinions about financial parameters. You may be on the same wavelength, or you may be on different bandwidths completely. But each needs to hear the other spouse speak. Foster communication at every step in your joint battle against infertility. Money matters are no exception. After looking at your current financial situation, what does each partner feel is the limit on what should be spent on infertility treatments? Maybe it's a percentage of your monthly income. Maybe it's a particular chunk of your savings account.

*After trying several months of infertility treatments, we decided that our money would best be spent helping a child who had already been born versus spending the money trying to conceive.*
*—Brian and Shelli*

*Establish a rough estimate of the cost of each level of treatment.* Talk with your fertility specialist about a possible scenario of treatment for you and your spouse. Then talk with someone in the doctor's business office to obtain accurate figures on what those procedures cost. Find out *ahead of time* what your insurance company will cover and what it won't. Otherwise, you'll probably have a fainting spell by the mailbox one day when you get the bill for your portion of the treatment. Expect to be shocked by the costs.

Ignorance is not bliss in this respect. As emotionally volatile as this struggle is, you need to look at the cold, hard, financial facts before you jump into the deep end of the fertility treatment pool. The deeper you go into infertility procedures, the quicker the costs escalate. It's common to repeat a procedure several times before success is reached or before moving on to more intricate treatments. Expect to pay for *more than one* of each procedure. Budget accordingly and draw your boundaries.

*At what point financially will you know it's time to stop pursuing treatments?* Assuming you don't achieve pregnancy and a live birth, how will you know it's time to stop going for one more round of treatment? Will it be when the money runs out? Will it be when you exhaust the amount you previously set aside? It's better to know beforehand where you stop and go no further, rather than to let circumstances (lack of money) control your stopping point.

It's a matter of feeling in control of your destiny. If you know where and when you will stop, *you* are the one in control. If you let your starving bank account determine your limits, then something else is controlling your options. So much about infertility is out of your control. If you can be in control of how much you spend, then you're regaining some command over the problem.

*We started with six months of Clomid, with the last three months including insemination. Then we did two cycles of Pergonal with insemination, after which our doctor wanted to do gamete intrafallopian transfer (GIFT). It wasn't covered by our insurance company, and we had decided to stop fertility treatments when our insurance no longer covered the procedures. We spent on adoption the $10,000 that GIFT would have cost.* —*Joy and Jeff*

*What options will you want to consider if you can't attain a live birth?* After the specialists have done all they can do, or when you reach your predetermined stopping point, what will you do if you're still childless? What options will interest you? Domestic adoption through an adoption agency? Private adoption? International adoption? Fostering? Will you decide to be child-free?

Try to keep a little of your savings on a back burner for the choice(s) that may interest you. Most couples can't pursue pricey IVF *and* still have all the needed funds for adoption expenses, but you can at least explore what some of the base costs will be. Some agencies have payment plans after you've made an initial down payment.

The National Adoption Information Clearinghouse (NAIC) Web site has a helpful document entitled "Cost of Adopting," which provides average adoption costs for domestic and international adoptions, plus adoption benefits, subsidies, or loan options. (To view online or download, go to www.calib.com/naic/ and look through the document list for "Cost of Adopting.")

When I walk through our neighborhood, there's one house I always dread approaching. The owner stands out on the front lawn to smoke and lets his dogs roam the yard unleashed. One dog is small, but the other dog is big and lean. I'm not convinced his bark is worse than his bite. As I approach, the dogs run to the very edge of the yard, barking and yelping, and I consider finding refuge on top of the nearest parked car. Though my heart races every time, I've never seen the dogs go past the invisible boundary that the owner has trained them to observe. The boundaries aren't there to punish the dogs, but to protect them from traffic and from hurting panicked passers-by like me.

If you'll take the time right now to prayerfully determine where you want to draw your boundary lines in the Valley of Infertility, you'll find that when you reach them, you won't feel punished, but protected. You'll feel more in control of your destiny because you've set limits for yourself based on what your goals are for your future.

*Jody and Marvin*
## Financial choices

Marvin was thirty-six and Jody was thirty-five when they married. "We had no reason to delay the process of starting a family, considering our ages," Jody said, so they quickly started fertility treatments.

Jody knew she had fertility problems because she and her first husband, Rick, had battled it during what should have been her most fertile years. She married soon after she graduated from high school, and by age twenty-one she had turned to the doctors for help in getting pregnant. "But we could never produce a pregnancy at all," she said. Then, when Jody was thirty-one, her life changed forever when Rick was killed in an automobile accident. Devastated, Jody worked hard to put her life back together. She went to college, graduated, and became an occupational therapist.

Several years later at a church Christmas party for single adults, Jody met Marvin. After they married they started the basic infertility treatments. Less expensive procedures like insemination didn't bring pregnancy, so they gathered their resources to spend the big bucks on in-vitro fertilization (IVF). At the same time, Marvin and Jody were drawing up house plans for their dream home. This was no mansion on a golf course, but a modest home on a quiet, country road where Marvin's family had owned land for years. They saved money by living in a mobile home on Marvin's land. But now it was time to begin building. Or was it?

The couple came to a crossroads—a new home or a baby? They didn't have to question for long—their desire for a family far exceeded their need for a dream home. They used their savings to continue infertility treatments.

The first round of injections to boost Jody's egg production in preparation for IVF resulted in only three eggs, and of those only one fertilized embryo survived. Jody's eggs just weren't surviving long after fertilization. That one embryo was implanted, but it didn't survive. She never had any indication that she was pregnant. "I lucked out in that our insurance covered most of the medications," Jody remembers. "But the cost of the clinic's involvement was not covered." Each IVF procedure cost $8,000 to $10,000. They could afford only one more round. Surely this would be the one that worked.

Jody and Marvin have a vibrant faith. And through all the praying, asking, requesting, and waiting, they believed the second IVF would be successful. When the fertility shots produced seven eggs, they were thrilled. But only one egg grew well in the lab. The implantation worked, and within weeks Jody began feeling the wonderful abnormalities that infertile women long for—bloating, nausea, and queasiness. At her doctor's recommendation she took time off from work to rest so that the pregnancy would be protected. She began planning to adjust her work in order to keep from having to lift heavy patients.

"I really believed God was going to give us this child," Jody says. "I just felt it was meant to be. The Lord had protected that one little embryo, and everything felt so right."

But between her eighth and tenth week Jody began spotting. Her miscarriage was confirmed by her doctor soon after. Although the fertility clinic they'd worked with had been extremely accommodating on the financial end, the couple was simply out of money for more IVF procedures. Reality was settling upon them in waves—an unlimited number of IVFs might never provide a live birth if Jody's eggs were not healthy and able to survive.

"My eggs basically were getting old. They just weren't viable," she says.

They moved on to consider a donor egg. "The cost was a big consideration, probably $10,000 to $12,000, plus our insurance wouldn't cover these medications," Jody says. "And what if it still didn't work? What if I still couldn't carry a baby to term? We realized that we had to face the truth. The additional cost of a donor procedure just wasn't feasible; plus there was the fear of another failure."

"I wanted to give Marvin a biological child," Jody says. "I wanted to be able to pass on his genes. He is such a wonderful person, and I knew his genes would make a wonderful child. I don't know how much of the qualities passed down are nature or nurture; but for him, for his family, I wanted to give him a child of his own." Marvin regularly tried to talk Jody out of being so concerned about giving his family a biological child. "He would tell me, 'This is just between us. The rest doesn't matter. We can't help it if we can't make a baby.'"

Had they considered adoption? It was a possibility they discussed; but after extensive fertility treatments, they didn't have money for an adoption agency fee.

However, another part of this story was quietly developing during the IVF procedures. For about three months Marvin and Jody had been giving almost daily childcare to a little girl and her baby brother who were in the custody of their grandmother. The grandmother worked two jobs to cover expenses, and she was thankful Jody and Marvin volunteered to watch the children for free. Eventually, the kids went to church with them on Sunday mornings and Wednesday nights and became a part of every aspect of their lives. They helped the girl with her homework every night. They bathed the kids and put them to bed for a few hours before their grandmother picked them up when she got off work after 11:00 P.M. When the baby boy turned one year old, Marvin and Jody gladly hosted the birthday party at their house.

Jody commented that getting to enjoy the boy's infancy was "a special gift from God." And the little girl was glued to Marvin's side as soon as he came home from work. She helped him with the garden, the outdoor chores, and other adventures.

In a God-ordained turn of events, the grandmother decided that Jody and Marvin were the kind of parents that her grandchildren needed. The adoption of both children is currently under way. By waiting on God's timing and being available to love the children God had already put in their lives, Jody and Marvin found themselves with two children who were as "precious as any we could have given birth to. We just grew into a family."

# Chapter 8

# Surviving Holidays and Social Events

*Be prepared to face some of your toughest times around the holidays.*
*What makes it even more painful is the realization that, typically, so*
*many of our happiest memories are from holidays in our past.*

*—Edward*

Year after year, my heart told my head, *Here's another*
*Christmas with no children's stockings to hang on the mantle.* My
heart kept copious notes on matters like this, while my head
hoped to ignore these painful details and simply survive the
event. Another birthday would slip by. Then one of the toughest holidays of all—Mother's Day.

If you have a history of battling infertility, you could write
this chapter from the aching saga of your own journey, with a
long list of holiday horror stories. But if you're a novice in the
infertility war, the following pages give an overview of what
many people experience when holidays roll around. Is this
meant to plant seeds of fear? No. But if, during a holiday get-
together, you begin to feel something erupt from deep in your
heart, maybe one of the coping ideas in this chapter will help
you maintain your emotional equilibrium until you find a safe
haven to release your sadness. Knowing what to expect and
how to navigate the uneven terrain ahead helps us handle the
emotions we encounter.

## Remember how much you are loved

Family events are supposed to be times of happiness, lots of
conversation, food, and catching up on each other's lives.
(Joviality isn't too high on your priority list these days, is it?)
The truth is, some of these holidays and family gatherings

simply need to be lived through, putting forward the best face you can muster. Remember these are the people you love and who have loved you since you were the one in diapers. Though they may not understand your grief, they deserve to share in your life right now. And you need to be part of their lives too. You are a valuable person to the Lord and to your family. Infertility does not undermine your worth. You still have much to share—your smile, your hugs, your warmth, and your love.

You may need to look Cousin Helen straight in the eye and tell her sincerely, "Even though we're running into all kinds of roadblocks as we try to have a baby, I just want you to know that I am sincerely thankful your pregnancy is going well. Tell you what, let's pray for each other in the coming months. I'll pray for your safe pregnancy and you pray that God will give us a child soon." You don't have to say you're *happy* she's pregnant with her fourth child—happy and thankful are mutually independent feelings. You can still be *thankful* for her and her baby's health without feeling the need to be gushy and over-the-top with your comments.

### Confide with caution

Some families are open books where everyone knows the minutiae of everyone's lives. Aunt Peggy's colostomy bag is talked about as easily as the fresh coat of paint Uncle Mark put on the shed. Families like this are prone to dish out tomes of homespun advice on how to get pregnant. Just how much can you stomach in one sitting? Listen as long as you feel you can, then brightly ask for a new subject. "I can only remember so much advice; and if we keep it up, I'll have to start taking notes!"

Then there are families who don't talk about anything personal. A friend told me that her family was so private, they would sit in the same room and watch a hilarious sit-com, but no one laughed aloud. While your infertility issues are not kitchen-table talk, the flip side is that your pain is ignored because it is either unknown or off-limits.

It helps to feel acknowledged as you walk through infertility. With nephews and nieces romping around, you feel lost and alone among people who share your common history.

Have you always felt that way or has infertility changed how you feel around your family? Most couples admit the latter—your thwarted quest for parenthood has made you feel like you don't belong.

Consider taking at least one person aside and confiding in them as much as you feel comfortable. Find someone who has been your cheerleader through the years, someone you know well, perhaps someone who has experienced infertility in the past or has suffered through another kind of grief.

Great-aunt Sadie may not understand the nuances of current infertility technology, but she knows what it's like to hurt and long for something to be different. Maybe you can tell her, "This ordeal is difficult for us; and even though there's nothing you can do to make it right, it makes me feel better just knowing that you're now aware of what we're going through. You don't have to tell anyone else in the family, but it'll make me feel better just to know that when I meet your glance across the room, you'll understand what's going on in my heart." Keep her updated periodically, and Aunt Sadie will be sharing an extra measure of your joy when you become parents.

### Journal your feelings

Over the years, when I've felt the lousiest I haven't wanted to journal much. All those gray feelings swamped me—why would I want to wade through them again to put them on paper? The surprise has been that when I did journal my darkest hours, I found it a surprising outlet. Occasionally, sentences flowed out of my pen that I hadn't consciously figured out beforehand. Sometimes I found myself solving an emotional frustration simply by venting it on paper.

Write about why a particular event is making you grieve anew your lack of children. Did the snowfall that blanketed your home on Christmas Eve make you think about how incredible it would be to share that moment with your children, watching the flakes through a foggy window? Write about how you wanted to share that moment with your children, snuggled up in bulky sweaters and warm socks.

Those from-the-gut scribbles will speak powerfully to you in the years to come. They are a record of who you are at this moment in time, where you were in your struggle with infertility, what you were working for and dreaming about. Perhaps one day you can show your child how much he or she was hoped for, prayed for, and thought of, even while he or she was not yet born.

### Do some vicarious parenting

When the family reunion finds you trying to avoid getting drawn into another endless conversation, the old folks' game of dominoes isn't up your alley, and the dessert table would mean death to your waistline, find where the youngest children are hiding out.

Cousin Christy could enjoy a moment of relaxation as you cuddle her baby with a bottle. Find your three-year-old niece and offer to help her up and down the slide. A little fun and laughter will loosen the tight grip that grief has on your heart.

While you're at it, consider it "field research." What makes a baby stop crying? Does a seven-month-old have teeth? Take mental notes on how a three-year-old climbs a ladder. What is she scared of? How did you reassure her? What does she like to talk about? What letters does she not yet pronounce correctly? How far can she get with her ABCs and 123s? You have a lot of love in your heart for children. Until you have your own, don't squelch your gift of love by keeping it sealed up.

Now let's work our way through the calendar and look at the major holidays, as well as some survival tips for each.

### ◆ *Christmas*

Christmas is one of the toughest of all holidays for infertile couples. Our culture views Christmas as a holiday where children's fanciful dreams come to life. Our churches center observances around the birth of Baby Jesus to young, fertile Mary. Our families delight as the youngest in the clan crawls through discarded wrapping paper, boxes, and bows.

Meanwhile, your soul feels like it's caving in because it's yet another Christmas that a child's laughter (specifically, *your* child's laughter) won't reverberate off the walls. Another Christmas when an extra stocking won't be hung. Another

Christmas when you can't buy those adorable "Baby's First Christmas" ornaments or those little red and green outfits for infants and toddlers. Parents take their kids to sit on Santa's lap, but you're an observer, not a participant.

*I can imagine myself sitting by candlelight and telling my children—whose eyes are wide and innocent, whose angelic faces outshine every angel ornament on our tree—that God sent little Baby Jesus to be born in Bethlehem.*

—*my journal*

*Friends' Christmas cards arrived from all around the country, complete with pictures of their growing families. It only reemphasized that all our friends, maybe even the whole world, seemed to have children—everyone except us.*

—*Lou Ann*

### Survival tips

**1. Focus on the spiritual meaning of Christmas.** Instead of trying to avoid Christmas and/or children completely (good luck!), nurture your soul with the wonder of God's gift to mankind. Observe Advent in your home with your spouse. For your quiet times, assign yourself a mini-research project of finding all the prophetic references to the coming Christ in the Old Testament and write them in a book that can be referred to every year at Christmas. Memorize Luke 2:1–20, and hold the Christmas story in your heart.

**2. Write down your childhood Christmas memories.** Buy a journal or start a scrapbook of everything you can remember from Christmases you and your spouse experienced as children. What were your family traditions? Think of things you will want to do with your own children one day. How can you make Christ the central aspect of your celebrations?

Go one step further and include pictures from past Christmases. Dig around in your mom's and mother-in-law's closets for old photos. Ask older family members (parents, grandparents, aunts, uncles) for input about what went on during family get-togethers, too. They can probably remember some of your childhood stunts you've forgotten about!

**3. *Give a part of yourself to others at Christmas.*** You might think that avoiding people altogether would be the best thing to do, but you would be shortchanging yourself. So many people need your love at Christmas. Many communities or churches sponsor an Angel Tree—a way for people to buy specific gifts for children whose parents are in prison. Food pantries, homeless shelters, and charities have many needs at Christmas—both monetary and "elbow grease." Pick one that you will do this season.

**4. *Help an unfortunate child have a better Christmas.*** Remember that many, many children don't have the stereo-typical holiday we find in Christmas ads: No toasty fireplace, no stack of gifts on Christmas morning, no cookie- and candy-making messes in a warm kitchen. Is there a children's hospital in your area? Call the hospital and ask for ways you can help make Christmas brighter for a child—maybe buying a gift or helping with a party.

Does your community have a children's home or orphanage? You don't have to think twice to know there will be needs there.

**5. *Create memories with a special child in your life.*** Even though you want to be creating memories with *your* child, think about spending time with someone else's child. Offer to baby-sit for the evening while the parents go Christmas shopping. Think of an age-appropriate activity to do with the child, maybe something you'd like to do with your child one day. Children like to surprise their parents, so even helping them make a homemade Christmas card can be an adventure. With an inkpad, a child can put her handprint on paper and create a treasure her parents will appreciate. And if the activity doesn't go off as smoothly as you expected, that's perfectly normal.

One Christmas, I baby-sat Alexander, my two-year-old nephew, while his parents attended a church party. I had planned a secret candy-making party for just the two of us. We made chocolate-covered pretzels and white chocolate with peppermint sprinkles. He was delighted to help cook something for his mommy and daddy—and he was eager to help wrap the goodies in colorful plastic and hide the bundles under their Christmas tree. I took pictures of the whole ordeal and later made Alexander a simple picture book to help him remember our very exclusive party. Just recently, I saw the book among his toys and began looking at it. He immediately said, "I remember that! You and I made candy one night for Mom and Dad."

**6. Limit your social engagements.** Decline party invitations where you'll be surrounded by children, or just limit your party participation altogether. Sometimes attending adult parties can be just as exhausting—so many conversations include long updates on everyone's kids. You're not being Grinch-ish, just realistic in what you can expect of yourself right now. Attend the Christmas Eve service that's least likely to attract parents with young children, such as one at midnight. Avoid crowded malls and stores by shopping from catalogs or online.

### ◆ Mother's Day and Father's Day

If Christmas is hard because of its obvious family overtones, then these two holidays are like bombs being dropped on your life. While everyone is celebrating the women who are mothers and the men who are fathers, you and your spouse feel severely cheated . . . again.

Churches ask mothers to stand in the congregation and be recognized. Some churches honor the oldest mother, the newest mother (she's your age; or worse, she's younger), the mother with the most children (while you're thinking, *Hey, God, all I'm asking for is* one!), but never do they acknowledge those who crave motherhood.

We were members of a church that had baby dedication on Mother's Day. A whole line of squirming babies, complete with happy parents (trying in vain to minimize the squirming), stood before the amused church family. Laughter trickled through the crowd as one little guy wanted to slobber on the pastor's microphone. All the parents were our peers or younger—they had children, why couldn't we? Edward and I sat stunned and expressionless. Our hearts felt drained again.

*At a Mother's Day recognition service in our church, we noticed that every female friend sitting within three rows of us stood in response to the pastor's call for mothers to be recognized. Among them was a fifteen-year-old girl that we'd worked with in the community. There she was with her tummy full of baby. Our hearts sank, and the "Why?" questions began.*      —*Dinah and Keith*

*I wish people would realize how horrible it feels on Mother's Day to be a woman who has miscarried and has never been able to bring a child to term. I'm a mother too! But because I don't have any living children, I'm not considered a "real" mother.*      —*Kelly*

Father's Day doesn't have quite the ordeal made over it, but men who want to be dads are no less earnest in their desire to nurture a child. Father's Day can be just as painful to them as Mother's Day is for women. Men who want to be fathers need to be recognized, too.

*Father's Day just brought to the forefront the fact that I wasn't a father. It drove home the point like a knife straight to my heart. Would I ever become one? The longer we traveled this road, the more painful it became. I remember the first year it was just a twinge of pain as I sat in the Father's Day recognition service. But as the years went by, the pain became so intense that we eventually avoided going to church at all on Father's Day.*      —*Edward*

Making it through these two holidays is tough. Thankfully, they don't occupy a whole season like Christmas does.

### Survival tips

**1. *Turn your focus to your parents and others.*** Rather than zeroing in on their own lack of motherhood or fatherhood, many infertile couples focus completely on their own parents or those who've been like parents. Find new and meaningful ways to honor these people who have invested so much in your life. Was there a particular Sunday School teacher who was a lighthouse during the storms of your adolescence? Did your third-grade teacher make you feel especially loved the first day you returned to school after the funeral of your favorite grandmother? What about the youth director who told you funny jokes at the hospital while your leg was set in a cast after you broke it on the ski slopes?

Like the account we find in Luke 17:11–19, only one man in ten returned to thank Jesus for healing him of leprosy. You may have expressed your gratitude to these people in earlier years, but think how incredible it would be for that person to realize that you still remember his or her act of kindness.

**2. Avoid the prefab greeting cards.** Do yourself a favor and don't stand at a greeting card display searching for a card for your parents. It can really do a number on you to see all the cards *you* might receive if you were a parent. Do something different: Write a letter thanking your parents for specific things they did in raising you. Recall particular times of family fun or recount a memorable lesson you learned. Or get creative and make a card. Your parents will treasure it just as much as the cards you made as a child.

**3. Don't give up on church altogether.** You don't have to be sitting on a church pew to honor God's admonition that we "not give up meeting together" (Heb. 10:25). God has an uncanny way of blessing us simply for being there. Serve that Sunday in another area of the church. Assemble bulletins for the next service. Count the offering money or sort the visitors' cards. Tag along in the bus ministry. Spend that time in the church's prayer room, interceding for the needs listed there.

Some women don't mind being around other people's children, but just don't want to endure a Mother's Day recognition service that they can't be part of. If that's you, then volunteer for children's church or the church nursery. Several women told me they enjoy rocking babies in the nursery. If you know your emotional boundaries, you'll know if a stint in the nursery would do you more harm than good.

◆ *Birthdays and Anniversaries*
Nobody puts much stock in making wishes as you blow out your birthday candles; but just in case there was some merit to it, I wished for a baby on several birthdays. (I also wished on that occasional falling star.)

Birthdays are your personal milestones in life. As each one passes, you realize it's another milestone you're not sharing with your child. Will your child even know you as a *young* person? Will your child remember you in your twenties? Thirties? Forties? You worry about whether you'll have enough adulthood left to enjoy watching your child grow up.

Your wedding anniversary is another doozy. Even though you know you should celebrate your union, you can't get away from the fact that the union can't seem to produce a child. The very fact that a wedding anniversary marks the coming together of two people can painfully remind you that when you exchanged your vows, you had no inkling that an infertility battle was lying in wait.

Infertility casts a long shadow over anniversaries and birthdays, but it doesn't have to leave them in complete darkness. These events mark personal times of *your* life, so give yourself permission to be consciously nice to yourself, even though the old self-esteem may be in the dumps.

## Survival tips

*1. Recognize the good things you've done in your life.* Realize how many people you've touched through your ministry.

*2. Be kind to yourselves.* On your birthday or anniversary, treat yourselves to some pampering—his and her massages or even just your favorite flavors of ice cream. Watch a favorite movie. Think about the great memories you've shared. By the way, does anyone ever really watch their wedding video? Do it this year!

*3. Find one new thing to do together.* What new memories can you make? As unbelievable as it seems, the time you have together now will be hard to come by once parenthood walks through your door. You'll long for time alone with your spouse. Use this time wisely to build a stronger marriage, to set and reach goals for your spiritual lives, to explore your abilities and gifts in full. Now is the time to take a missions trip together and serve in another state or country. Ask God to show you how to use this time wisely.

**4. Nurture your marriage above all else.** Find ways to help each other through the holidays by intentionally talking about how you feel. One spouse may not want to share much, but both of you need to talk about how you're feeling. Both need to hear how the other is feeling. (See chapter 4, "Marriage: Will Yours Survive or Thrive?") Maybe this is the Thanksgiving to take that weekend ski trip you've always dreamed about. Sure, you'll miss out on the grand spread of food with your relatives, but you both need to decide if missing out is worse than encountering the social pain. And remember, this avoidance behavior isn't forever. Maybe it's just this year's holiday that you need a breather from.

#### ◆ Halloween and Fall Festivals

While I was growing up, Halloween was laced with simple traditions at my house. We always ate corn chip–chili pies on Halloween night before we went trick-or-treating. My brother Ted always helped Dad carve the pumpkin. Mom used the same 1960s-era candy tray each Halloween. Pictures were always taken by the front door of me, Ted, and Cousin Sara in our costumed garb. The night always ended by going to Grandma's house to give her a private viewing of our Halloween costumes—and to receive a hefty addition to our candy bags.

I looked forward to sharing Halloween with my child. But when parenthood continued to elude us, just seeing children's costumes in the store would bring another wave of pain. I never knew whether I should buy a bag of candy to distribute because when Halloween arrived, I might be too bummed to look at an endless bevy of costumed children from the neighborhood. Sometimes I'd turn off all the lights and watch TV in the dark, just so no one would venture to ring our doorbell. Some years I felt stronger and could face the kids.

At its best, Halloween and fall festival events give families a chance to let children dress up and create fun memories. The popularity of safe events like church-sponsored festivals and community fairs affirm and undergird the "familyness" of late October. And when you're beating the bushes trying to start a family, you realize not a season passes when you don't feel the empty places in your heart.

## Survival tips

*1. Get to know your neighbors.* With an array of children at your doorstep all evening, why not use trick-or-treating as a time to pass along a word of Truth and Light? Stand on the porch and greet your neighbors as they walk by. One year, I wrapped a Bible verse around each piece of candy I distributed, praying that its truth would sink into the hearts of the children and their parents. Since then, I've seen colorful tracts for Halloween that explain God's love. Make your house a bright, safe beacon on a dark night.

*2. Carry on some of your childhood traditions.* One year it dawned on me that I didn't have to wait until we had children to make corn chip-chili pies on Halloween night. So I did it, just for us. It brought forth warm memories of my own childhood, of a time when words like *infertility* and *childlessness* weren't in my vocabulary. For fun, dig out old pictures of you and your siblings in your Halloween costumes.

*3. Focus on your friends.* Host a couples-only costume party. It's really a lot of fun to plan costumes as a couple. Plan it for a night after Halloween is over, when the candy, pumpkins, and costumes are all marked down drastically! Bob for apples, juggle tiny pumpkins, or make caramel-and-nut-covered apples on a stick.

◆ *Baby Showers*
Pure torture . . . don't you agree? Baby showers hit us where it hurts the most. One woman said that by attending a two-hour baby shower, she could completely unravel all the emotional balance God had helped her achieve in a month.

*The worst time was when I hosted a baby shower for a very good friend. It seemed that everyone there already had a baby or was getting ready to have one. I smiled all the way through it; but when I got home, Jeff asked me how it went. In frustration, I threw everything I was holding against the wall. From that day on, I didn't go to any baby showers until after we adopted our son.* —Joy

I remember sitting at the baby shower of a young woman who was at least a decade younger than I. She had been married only about a year and had gotten pregnant with absolutely no problem. I was miserable—trying to stay pleasant on the outside while crashing on the inside.

## Survival tips

**1. Send a gift.** For all but your very closest friends/relatives, just send a gift to a shower and skip attending it. And speaking of gifts, give a gift certificate rather than spend difficult moments searching the baby aisles for the perfect gift. Pick a store that sells baby merchandise and buy a gift certificate at any register, rather than buying it *in* the baby department.

**2. Don't host a shower for a while.** This can emotionally sabotage you for weeks. We wouldn't expect a new widow to sing at a wedding, would we? Likewise, set the limits of what you can reasonably expect of yourself.

**3. Determine how to cope if you must attend.** Let's say your sister is having her firstborn, and you really should be at the shower; plus you love her and want to. First, be as prayed-up as possible. You owe it to yourself to be in tune with your Lord and to fully claim His peace.

Second, at the event, focus on something besides the baby. Pray for the mother-to-be as she opens the gifts. Pray for her health, for her spiritual walk, for her new role as a mother, for her marriage, for the job she's leaving or taking time off from, for the time complications that will surely result.

Third, plan a definite arrival and departure time. Staying until the very end can be exhausting. Give yourself a pre-planned excuse. Plan something with your husband that will require you to leave a little early.

Finally, before you get there, plan what you'll do if you find yourself emotionally overwhelmed. Determine that you'll let your tears flow when you're in the safety of your own car or at home. A quick trip to the bathroom or to the kitchen for another cup of punch may be the breather you need to keep your tears in check and your emotions at bay during the shower. There's nothing wrong with feeling the way you do about your infertility, but remember that this event is a high-light for the mother-to-be. You'd feel terrible if one day some-one broke down at *your* baby shower, wouldn't you? Let your greatest gift be your support and genuine concern for her on this day.

◆ *Other Holidays and Annual Events*
Our calendars are sprinkled with annual events that are meaningful to us in varying degrees—New Year's Day, Valentine's Day, the Fourth of July, family reunions, Thanksgiving, the beginning and ending of school. The ten-dency is to look at *any* holiday and say, "Here's another _____ and still I have no children to share it with. This time last year, I thought for sure we'd be parents by the time _____ rolled around again."

The key is to find a way to experience these holidays with-out focusing on how infertility is ruining it for you.

**Survival tip**

*Make it special for someone.* If you could, how would you share this event with your child? How would you prepare? What would you do? Where would you go? Keep a list of ideas in your journal for all the things you want to do with your child one day. But you don't have to wait until God blesses you with a child to share yourself with others, even with other children. Consider these ideas as ways to reach out on special days with the love of Christ.

•Take a friend to the Valentine's Day brunch at a local restaurant.

•Ask your unchurched neighbors and their children to join you for a Fourth of July picnic and community fireworks.

•Put together a bag of goodies to congratulate a co-worker's child for finishing the school year with flying colors.

•Volunteer at a soup kitchen on Thanksgiving Day.

•Buy some new school clothes for a child and give the clothes to a local ministry that helps families in need. (Ministries get used clothes all the time. New clothes will be a treat to the receiver.)

These activities can help you weather infertility's storms as God directs you in His plan for how and when you'll parent. Don't try to live as a hermit and avoid all potential pain from social events. God has given you the gift of life—*your life.* He wants you to use these days and events to know Him better and to share His love with others. As you survive holidays and special times in the midst of longing to fulfill the role of parent, look for ways to fulfill the first role that God has called you to—the role of His disciple and the bearer of His love.

# Chapter 9

# Infertility Treatments, Meds, and Tips

*After months of trying, we've come to the conclusion that pregnancy isn't going to "just happen" for us. We know very little about infertility and haven't found much information out there. What I have found is a lot of medical-speak, with regimented time frames and treatments, but not much from people who have been through this experience. I'm looking for information about the personal side of dealing with infertility. It would be nice to know that my frustration is valid (and normal), and how others have gotten through it.*

*—Nina*

If someone developed a board game based on infertility treatments, you'd land on spaces called "Timed Intercourse" or "Hormone Therapy," but you'd draw cards that read, "Sorry, you missed ovulation. Go back three spaces." If you're lucky, you'll draw a card that reads, "Go directly to pregnancy, but pay another $7,000." You'd win when you landed on "Healthy Delivery."

Infertility isn't a game at all, but rather an experience of faith, strategy, skill, persistence, and a little bit of chance thrown in. And once in a while you may feel like a token being pushed from one space to the next.

If you're new to the infertility journey, then the terms and procedures thrown at you can be completely confusing and overwhelming. This chapter gives a basic explanation of the general route you might take through infertility, explaining which tests usually precede others and what happens at the various levels of treatment.

Also, some of our survey participants have contributed their memories of what they felt like on various medications.

Keep in mind that no one can expect to feel wonderful when taking these meds! Their responses can be a little overwhelming to the couple just starting their infertility investigation. I include these comments not to scare you away, but to give you an idea of what other women have experienced. At least you won't be caught off guard, as they were.

This chapter partners with the glossary in the back of this book. You'll may want to refer to the glossary as you read this chapter, to acquaint yourself with the lingo.

Volumes of information exist on infertility and how to solve it. It would be impossible to provide everything you ever wanted to know about infertility technology in this one chapter. But using this information as a basis of understanding, you can expand your knowledge by going to the Web sites listed under "Resources" at the end of the book. Your doctor can also tell you about new procedures being developed.

### Understanding the problem

• Infertility affects 6.1 million US women and their partners, or about 10 percent of the reproductive-age population.

• In about 40 percent of infertile couples, the male partner is either the sole cause or a contributing cause of infertility.

• Female infertility problems break down as follows: Twenty-five percent have irregular/abnormal ovulation. Thirty-five percent have tubal blockage and/or peritoneal factors. Thirty-five percent of the women who have a laparoscopy have endometriosis.

• About 20 percent of couples who do a complete diagnostic work-up are diagnosed with unexplained infertility because no specific cause is identified.

• More than 70,000 babies have been born in the US as a result of assisted reproductive technology (ART). About 45,000 of these births are specifically credited to in vitro fertilization (IVF).

• In vitro fertilization and similar treatments account for less than 5 percent of infertility services, and only three-hundredths of 1 percent (.003) of US health care costs. *(Statistics from the American Society for Reproductive Medicine)*

• The World Health Organization (WHO) estimates that approximately 8- to 10 percent of couples experience some form of infertility problem. On a worldwide scale, this means that 50 to 80 million people suffer from infertility. However, the incidence of infertility may vary from region to region. In France, 18 percent of couples of childbearing age said that they had difficulties in conceiving.

• *Primary infertility* is the inability to become pregnant after a year of regular, unprotected intercourse. *Secondary infertility* refers to a couple who has birthed a child but cannot bring about pregnancy (or the live birth) of a second child.

### Diagnostic measures

Your doctor is a lot like Sherlock Holmes. Each case is different, each is a mystery, and each requires great attention to detail. Not all the following diagnostic tests are required for every woman, but as additional concerns arise or as pregnancy continues to be elusive, more tests will be performed. The treatment plan is tailored for each couple's specific needs. Remember that no one has the precise medical history that you do. Your doctor's goal is for you to get pregnant using the least-invasive, least-complicated means possible.

After a year of unprotected, frequent (two to three times per week) intercourse, a couple should get pregnant on their own. Any longer than that with no pregnancy, and it's time for intervention. But by the time you give up trying to get pregnant on your own and head to the doctor, you're ready to make some fast progress. He or she will insist on these diagnostic measures to assess what's going on inside you and your spouse. It may seem slow and laborious, but it's what we all went through. Both partners will probably undergo physical exams. Bring your medical records with you to save time having to request them from your other doctors.

As for testing, men don't have nearly as many hoops to jump through; but when you think about it, a woman's reproductive system is a complex system. It not only produces the egg, but provides an environment for it to be fertilized, a location in which the embryo will grow, a feeding system that nurtures the baby, and a delivery system that births the child.

The InterNational Council on Infertility Information Dissemination (INCIID; pronounced like the word *inside*) recommends tracking the length of your menstrual cycles for several months before your first appointment, as well as charting your basal body temperature, just to give your doctor some preliminary information. INCIID also recommends using ovulation predictor tests and recording the results.

*Tests for her:* The first goal is to make sure the woman is ovulating, and when. This can be determined through *ovulation prediction kits, basal body temperature charts, blood tests* to evaluate her estrogen and progesterone levels, and by *endometrial biopsy.*

A *hysterosalpingogram* (HSG) studies a woman's fallopian tubes and uterus. A laparoscopy can assess and remove endometriosis. A *postcoital test* detects sperm-mucus interaction problems, the presence of sperm antibodies, and the quality of the cervical mucus. An *endometrial biopsy* samples the endometrium late in the reproductive cycle to determine whether ovulation has occurred and if the endometrium is developing properly. A *hysteroscopy* examines the uterus to determine why a woman experiences recurring pregnancy loss. *Blood tests* check for hormone levels: An androgen panel looks for levels of free testosterone and dihydroeprandrostone (DHEAS); other tests monitor prolactin, progesterone, thyroid- stimulating hormone (TSH), free T3, free thyroxine (T4), total testosterone, free testosterone, and androstenedione. *Ultrasound exams* assess the thickness of the endometrium, monitor follicle development, and the condition of uterus and ovaries.

*Test for him:* Semen analysis is the first test done to assess the man's reproductive health. This procedure checks the number of sperm he produces, as well as the health, motility (movement), and number of sperm. If there is a problem with sperm, that information will determine the next steps to make pregnancy more likely. For instance, to improve the sperm's odds of making a hit with the egg, it can be collected, washed, sorted, then injected directly into an egg (a process called Intracytoplasmic Sperm Injection or ICSI) or placed in close proximity to the egg (by In Vitro Fertilization—IVF, Gamete Intrafallopian Transfer—GIFT, or Zygote Intrafallopian Transfer—ZIFT) before implantation in the woman.

*Test for both partners:* The wife and husband may be required to have a Duke's test (an infection or antibody test) done on the cervical mucus or semen to look for signs of bacteria or antibodies that would attack the sperm. A man's body may produce antibodies against his own sperm, or a woman may produce antibodies against her husband's sperm. Both problems indicate a malfunction of the immune system since the sperm is seen as a disease-causing invader. Steroid therapy may suppress the antibodies, or the sperm might be washed prior to use in other procedures (Intrauterine Insemination— IUI, IVF, ICSI, etc.).

### Entry-level procedures and medications
*Timed intercourse:* The specialist may suggest trying an initial effort at making intercourse happen more frequently by paying closer attention to the woman's body temperature and ovulation cycles. This is an attempt to have the sperm in the Fallopian tube at the time the egg is released and begins to travel down the tube. An advanced version of this procedure includes an ultrasound to monitor follicular development and uterine lining. A "trigger shot" of human chorionic gonadotropin (HCG) can be given to spur ovulation and set up the timing for intercourse.

*Lupron:* Among other things, Lupron is used to help eliminate remaining endometriosis after laparoscopy has removed most of it. Anyone who's been on Lupron will tell you it's an early introduction to menopause—though you have no periods, you gain the privilege of experiencing hot flashes and mood swings. Lupron simulates menopause by shutting down estrogen production.

*Lupron always affected me a few days after I got the injection. It was as if a big black cloud would come over me. I would cry over the strangest things! One time my girlfriends and I went to a movie together, and they were talking about how chicken pox was going around with all their kids. I could barely get home before I was crying, "We don't have kids; we have dogs! My dogs will never have chicken pox. I can't take my dogs shopping. I'm missing out on so much!"*　　　　　　　　　　　　　　　　　　　　　　—*Ann*

## Midlevel options

Moving up the ladder of complexity, your doctor may include these measures in your fertility treatment plan:

*Hormone therapy:* Fertility drugs act on the glands that produce key hormones. One of the most common is clomiphene citrate (Clomid, Serophene). While a woman is taking it the ovaries are monitored by ultrasound to follow the development of follicles. During hormone therapy, couples will be instructed to have intercourse on specific days, or they will increase the likelihood of getting sperm closer to the egg by doing intrauterine inseminations (IUI). The most common side effects of clomiphene citrate are headaches, nausea, vomiting, insomnia, hot flashes, bloating, abdominal pain, ovarian enlargement, nervousness, and visual disturbance.

Here are some comments from women who have taken fertility drugs.

*While I was on Clomid, I would go to work, sit at my desk, and at 2:00 every afternoon, I'd get up, walk around downtown, and just cry. Then I'd go back to my desk, sit down, and work the rest of the afternoon. I did this for three months!* —*Cindy H.*

*The biggest struggle in our marriage occurred when I was placed on fertility pills. Just having to time my cycle each month and having to "try to get pregnant" on that one day each month was very stressful. When the time came . . . neither of us would feel like it, but we knew we had to try. One of the main reasons I will not seek treatment again is because of how the drugs made me feel. I was on an emotional roller coaster 24 hours a day, 7 days a week!* —*Shelli*

*Clomid made me sweaty at night with hot flashes during the day. I was weepy all the time, or I could just as easily bite someone's head off for nothing. The moodiness reminded me of PMS. It was terrible. I took Clomid for ten months total, and the doctor credits Clomid with the one child we were able to have. But truly, I credit God for giving us Briley.* —*Celeste*

*Follicle-stimulating hormone (FSH) injections:* Examples include Humegon, Repronex, Follistim, Pergonal. These make a woman produce more eggs, and ultrasound monitoring is necessary to accurately time insemination after ovulation.

*Clomid didn't make me crazy, but Pergonal did. Jeff said he never knew how I was going to act. I was like Dr. Jekyll and Mr. Hyde.*
*—Joy*

*With Humegon, I had hot flashes, was moodier, and I felt I wasn't thinking as clearly. Fertinex gave me hot flashes and moodiness, and it made me feel a little crazy, like there was a madwoman inside me!*
*—Jody*

*I don't remember being too stressed during the actual time I was getting the injections, but I remember telling a friend, in retrospect, that after they were over that I really was on edge. I cried a lot between the time of the injections and the pregnancy test. It was very stressful getting the shot at the exact same time each day, and ultrasounds every other day were difficult to arrange, since we already had a four-year-old who needed childcare during my sonogram.*
*—Deana*

*Clomid and Pergonal both did me in! I had horrible crying spells and felt that a black cloud hovered over me. I was totally convinced no one cared at all, not even my closest friends and family. How could they? They hadn't been on these drugs!*
*—Rhonda*

**Artificial insemination:** Intrauterine insemination injects sperm directly into the uterus to get more sperm closer to the egg. Usually two to six cycles of FSH and IUI are tried before moving to more aggressive levels of treatment. Intratubal insemination (ITI) injects washed sperm directly into the fallopian tubes.

**Progesterone treatment:** Progesterone is the hormone responsible for maintaining a pregnancy by keeping the endometrium thick and viable for the fertilized egg. Some women are given supplemental progesterone because they have low progesterone levels, which make it difficult to sustain a pregnancy. It's available as a suppository, lozenge, or intramuscular injection. Several women in my survey noted that the injections were extremely painful, the single worst aspect of their infertility procedures. Side effects include tenderness of breasts, bloating, moodiness, and weight gain. For some women it can be even worse.

*I frequently felt hopeless while taking progesterone. I felt edgy and was capable of flying off the handle without a moment's notice. Besides mood swings, I noticed I had heavier periods. In my journal, I described feeling like I was riding a train in a big, dark tunnel with no light or end in sight. In some of the darkest valleys, I even had thoughts of suicide. I wouldn't have followed through with it because I wouldn't put my family through that grief and because I wouldn't want to reflect poorly on the cause of Christ, as if His grace and comfort weren't sufficient to overcome my despair. But the thoughts were there, and my journal chronicles the influence progesterone had on my mental well-being.* —Paula

## High-tech options
Not long ago, these techniques were considered cutting edge, but now they're available to anyone—well, anyone with mildly deep pockets. In a few years, more procedures will be added to this list as science fiction becomes reality.

*IVF-ET:* In vitro fertilization (IVF) used with embryo transfer (ET) seems extremely common today, though it accounts for less than 5 percent of all fertility treatments in the US, according to the American Society of Reproductive Medicine. In infertility circles, it's not unusual to know several couples who have used IVF. IVF-ET is an option for women who have damaged fallopian tubes or women whose husbands have problems with sperm. A woman's ovaries are stimulated to produce a sufficient number of eggs, the eggs are surgically removed from the ovary and mixed with sperm outside the body in a glass dish (not a test tube) for about forty hours. The eggs are then examined to see which ones have fertilized and begun to divide into cells. These embryos (some may be frozen at the couple's request) are then placed directly in the woman's uterus, bypassing the fallopian tubes completely.
*SPA:* Sperm penetration assay. This test is done prior to an IVF cycle to determine if the man's sperm are likely to be able

to penetrate a woman's eggs. The sperm are mixed with hamster eggs; and if few sperm are able to penetrate the hamster eggs, intracytoplasmic sperm injection (ICSI) will be needed to make sure the sperm are directly injected into the eggs prior to returning the eggs to the fallopian tubes.

*ICSI:* Intracytoplasmic sperm injection. A single sperm is directly injected into an egg using micromanipulation. For men with abnormalities of sperm motility, count, and morphology (the appearance of a sperm's head/tail), IVF with ICSI is considered an extremely successful therapy. ICSI is always used in conjunction with IVF because once the egg is fertilized, it must be returned to the woman's uterus. When a couple's infertility problems reside only with the woman, IVF is used; but if the man also has male factor infertility, then ICSI is combined with IVF to make sure the sperm and the egg are joined before implantation.

*IVFs made me crazy with a capital C! With each in vitro, the effects of the meds got worse and worse. We stopped after three failed in vitros.*
                                                                                *—Ann*

*GIFT:* Gamete intrafallopian transfer. Egg meets sperm in the natural environment of the Fallopian tubes.

*ZIFT:* Zygote intrafallopian transfer. Egg meets sperm in a petri dish in a lab. Fertilized eggs (embryos) are then moved to a fallopian tube where they can make their way to the uterus, hopefully, to settle in comfortably there. Couples who have unexplained infertility, sperm antibodies, male factor infertility, or older women trying to conceive can benefit most from ZIFT.

*FET:* Frozen embryo transfer, also called cryopreservation. Embryos are frozen for future use. This involves a special liquid nitrogen freezer. The embryos are stored until ready to use, then submersed in liquid nitrogen until they are thawed, and placed into the uterus. Not all embryos survive the process of freezing and thawing. A 50-percent survival rate is considered reasonable.

*Donor egg:* Also called donor oocyte. This kind of program can help infertile couples who have problems with viable eggs. Sometimes a woman's eggs are simply poor quality, few in quantity, or perhaps premature menopause has begun. Unfertilized eggs are retrieved from another woman (donor) who is willing to donate her eggs for this specific purpose. Eggs are retrieved as they would be for an IVF procedure, fertilized with the man's sperm, then injected into the infertile woman (recipient). The donor is compensated for her time and duress.

*Donor sperm:* For couples in which male factor infertility makes it impossible to use the husband's sperm, this option allows them to have a baby using the wife's egg and sperm donated anonymously. The couple can choose the criteria by which sperm are selected (i.e., the man's physical characteristics). Using donor sperm is much less expensive and less complicated than donor eggs.

*Surrogate parenting:* A procedure in which a woman carries a baby to term for a couple in which the woman is unable to carry one herself. The surrogate may or may not use her own eggs, depending on the situation. She is impregnated via artificial insemination. A host surrogate mother denotes a woman who bears a child who was conceived via IVF using the husband's sperm and wife's egg, thus the surrogate mother is completely out of the genetic picture. Surrogacy is one of the most shaky legal options available to infertile couples because emotional issues arise for the surrogate about visitation rights, parental rights, etc. In the most messy situations, the surrogate may decide she doesn't want to place the child for adoption when the child was conceived using the surrogate's egg.

### Choosing a clinic
Those who pursue fertility procedures and those who pursue adoption have similar anxieties when it comes to finding a safe, reputable group of professionals to affiliate with. When you begin to think about finding a fertility clinic, here are some questions to consider.

*Regarding the clinic:* How long has the clinic been around? Is it a member of the Society for Assisted Reproductive Technology (SART)? How many transfers do they do each month? What are the staff's credentials? What is the rate of live births in comparison to patients just beginning ART? Does the clinic have sufficient experience with your specific infertility problems (if it has been identified)? Does it have cryopreservation facilities? Ask if the clinic has a waiting list (and how long it is), and if they offer counseling. Ask for a list of all the costs that you might run into.

*Regarding embryos:* What is the policy on custody of embryos if one parent should die or the couple divorces? What does the clinic do with extra embryos not implanted?

*Regarding multiple births:* How many multiple births do they see each year?

*Questions to ask yourself:* What are your opinions about creating more embryos than you'll use in one cycle? What would you want to do with the extra embryos? How many eggs would you want to be fertilized or transferred in a cycle? What about freezing extra embryos for later use?

Find a clinic that has a good reputation with your friends. You need a clinic and a specialist who will listen to your desires and convictions as you are guided through the process. For example, if you don't feel it's ethically right to freeze embryos, stand your ground and insist that only the number of eggs should be harvested and fertilized that will be implanted. It's your choice, and while you don't have a lot of control over the broad picture of infertility, this is one area where you can exercise some command.

## Fertility drugs: A bite out of your wallet

My pharmacist friend, Bob, gave me several examples of the costs of fertility drugs. It's not for the faint of heart or wallet! One woman bought a one-month supply of fertility meds; and while she only had to cover her co-pay (total of $300), the insurance company picked up the rest—about $11,000—for one month! Another woman was in her eleventh month of treatment and had easily spent about $60,000 on meds. (Remember that these costs are meds only—no procedures, doctor fees, or tests.) A third couple racked up so many expenses that when the procedures finally produced a live birth, she had to put the new baby in day care and go to work just so they could begin to pay off the medical bills from getting the baby.

Depending on the protocol a particular specialist follows, a woman can be on a dizzying number of medications all at once. One woman was on eleven different medications in one month.

Some couples find they can save money in several ways. First, ask the doctor if he or she has any samples to help defray at least part of the cost. Second, mail-order pharmacies (usually found on the Internet) can offer lower prices because they control their overhead by ordering only what they need from the drug companies. Bob cautions that some drugs are temperature-sensitive; if your package from the mail-order company sits in the back of a delivery truck in the summer heat, it can render the drug less effective. Ask the company about how they ship temperature-sensitive meds. Finally, ask couples who've gone before you if they know of a reduced-cost pharmacy in the area that specializes in stocking fertility drugs.

**Suggestions from those who've been there**
Experience is the best teacher, so here are helpful hints compiled from couples who have walked through infertility treatments.

*1. Keep a notebook of medical notes and questions.* If you're starting your treatments soon, be prepared: You're going see a lot of new faces for a lot of reasons. After a while, it all gets mushy in your head, and you'll have trouble remembering what result went with which test. One of the best things I've ever done to organize our medical histories is to keep a small spiral notebook with notes jotted from every doctor appointment we have. I also list medications prescribed and our reactions to them. It has helped me immensely, as the years go by, when I've forgotten what drug I took way back when and whether I showed any sensitivities to it. During your months/years of infertility treatments, keep your notebook out so you can write questions you have between appointments, then refer to them at the next visit. Write down as much as possible during the appointment. Some women take a microcassette recorder to the appointment, just to be able to review later on what the doctor said. Staying organized gives you more sense of control and a better understanding of what you're going through and where you are.

**2. Take your spouse with you whenever possible.** Extra ears and extra eyes are always beneficial. Plus, the extra brain comes in handy for remembering information afterwards.

**3. Ask your doctor or pharmacist for a printout of any possible side effects on all medications.** Also ask your doctor for the most common side effects she has noticed.

*Metrodin worked quickly for us, and it didn't make me crazy. But I did gain weight quickly. Within two weeks, my clothes weren't fitting. I knew, even if I was pregnant, I wouldn't be outgrowing clothes that fast! I asked the nurse and doctor about side effects, and they offhandedly remarked that they'd seen patients gain up to ten pounds a day on Metrodin! That was a potential side effect that should have been mentioned from the beginning.* —Cindy H.

**4. Try not to compare yourself to the other couples who have gone through similar procedures.** Okay . . . easier said than done. There's a real temptation to build false hopes around the results that someone else got with a particular procedure. Try to remember that every couple is distinctly different.

Is it worth the financial cost, plus the emotional, spiritual, mental, and physical strain? Certainly! The arrival of a child is worth every second of a potential parent's efforts and worries. We live in an era with opportunities that barren Hannah and Elkanah couldn't have dreamed of. But we must balance that enthusiasm with the sober truth that not every couple can experience a live delivery, even with all the medical miracles available. Each couple must determine not *if* all this effort is worth it, but *how much* and *how long* they will push forward before moving to nonbirth options. No across-the-board answer exists.

When you and your spouse are equipped with knowledge of the medical processes and allied with a doctor you feel confident about, you'll be able to make wise choices that take you closer to your goal.

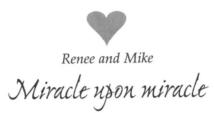

*Renee and Mike*

## Miracle upon miracle

When Renee and Mike watch their sons at play, they have every right to think of their sons as miracles two times over. First, their sons were conceived through ICSI and IVF procedures. But an additional level of wonder occurred when the one remaining embryo split and became identical twins.

After two miscarriages, Renee and Mike had tried most of the alphabetical options available at the time: GIFT, ZIFT, ICSI, IVF, and more IUIs than Renee cares to count! When they got to IVF, four embryos were implanted; but a later sonogram showed that only one survived. However, at the next sonogram two fetuses showed up on the screen. Her doctor was amazed: Identical twins occurring after implantation is extremely rare. Clark and Cole were born in 1995.

Did Renee and Mike set any emotional, financial, or physical boundaries to know when enough was enough? "Not really. We just kept trying," Renee remembers. "But we were nearing the end of what we could emotionally handle when I finally got pregnant. I'm not sure how much further we would have gone if the IVF hadn't been successful."

Renee learned a few things during her infertility journey. "First, educate the people around you. I gave informational pamphlets to my mother and close friends so they could understand what we were going through, and so they wouldn't ask or say the wrong things!"

Her next suggestion is to make sure the couple attends as many appointments together as possible. "Both of you are going through it, so you both need to be present."

# Chapter 10

# Adoption—God's Miraculous Tapestry

*Adoption is wonderful! I can't imagine loving a birth child any more than I love my adopted children. There are so many children who need parents who will love them. When they call you "Mama," it melts your heart and it doesn't matter if you carried them inside of you for nine months or not. That is your child! When God formed that child in the womb, it was your child. He is the One who puts families together!*

*—Katie*

Adoptive parents readily agree that adoption is an awe-inspiring unfolding of God's plans. With adoption, God moves not just a couple to adopt a child, but whole groups of people to participate in the creation of a new family. In our adoption of Ryan, five family units were orchestrated by God's hand to weave Ryan into our lives: A teenaged girl (1) became pregnant by her boyfriend (2); a Christian family (3) took her into their home; the birth mother and father finally agreed to an adoption plan; my husband's aunt and uncle (4) heard about the birth mother's plan; then they put us (5) in touch with the birth mother, who chose us to raise her child.

God is the Mighty Worker of intricate designs. Details that none of us could even imagine are intertwined with precise timing. Even the disappointments of infertility have their place in the miracle of adoption. God uses *everything*—our hurts and closed doors, our joys and hopes, our dreams—and creates an opportunity to welcome a child into our lives. God uses even our infertility to bring about the good things He has for us.

If you're afraid of stepping into the murky waters of adoption, I wish I could sit beside you and share with you the wonder that adoption has brought to our lives. It is *so far* from being a second-best option for having a family. We are now *thankful* that God allowed us to walk the road of infertility so that we would pursue adoption and become Ryan's parents.

Many couples would find this impossible to believe. It's not that we *enjoyed* infertility . . . who would? But now that we're on the other side of adoption and infertility (we're not trying to cure it any longer), that perspective makes sense. Granted, we didn't come to this opinion overnight, but after many years and many tears. If we'd birthed a child when we wanted to, if a dozen things had worked out when *we* wanted them to, we would never have been in the right place at the right time to take *this particular child* by adoption . . . a baby boy who, I firmly believe, had been destined since the beginning of time to be in our arms. God designed the tapestry for our family long, long ago. The threads are just now beginning to come together.

Not everyone comes to adoption with such openness. If you've set your heart completely on raising a child you birth, then the choice of adoption seems like second best, an option to be settled for, but certainly not "God's best" for your life. Maybe you don't think you could ever love someone else's child the way you would love your own flesh and blood. Maybe you don't like the factor of the unknown: What medical unknowns will this child bring into your family? Will she have learning disabilities? Has he inherited emotional deficiencies? Maybe you're afraid you'll get your heart stepped on if you set it out like a doormat.

You're certainly entitled to those feelings and opinions, but I hope you'll lay each one at God's throne and let Him direct you as to which concerns you should pick up again.

**But adoption seems so risky**
When you think of adoption, does your mind immediately fly to what you see on TV? Well, *that* can sure color your thinking! While I was writing this book, the news told of a messy adoption between birth parents in the US and adoptive parents in England that was reversed. A courtroom drama portrayed two birth parents fighting each other viciously for custody of their baby before finally giving him up for adoption. It's enough to scare anyone.

Infertility

*Don't take to heart all the horror stories you hear about adoption;
instead, seek out the positive stories. If I had only known then what
I know now, I would have adopted ten years earlier. It took only one
month from when we applied with the adoption agency until we had
our baby girl. The morning the birth mom went into labor, we called
everyone we knew and were blessed with prayer after prayer after
prayer. We were at the hospital when she was born, and we took her
home with us. When we got home our house was decorated in pink
and white. Everyone was waiting for us, with a stork in the front
yard that read "It's a girl!"*                       —Olaf and Linda*

The media practically never pushes happy adoption stories.
Why? Because it's not news. It's run-of-the-mill. An average
of 120,000 adoptions happen every year in the US, with less
than 0.1 of 1 percent ever contested. The *exception* to the rule
is when an adoption has a disastrous flavor to it. And the
more disastrous, the more the media pounces on it.

So what about the risk factor? Everything monumental in
life comes with risk. Marriage is risking that two people's
happiness together will outweigh their happiness as individuals. Taking on a new job and leaving another behind is risky.
Infertility treatments are loaded with risks; no clinic on earth
can absolutely guarantee a positive outcome. The impact of
fertility drugs on a woman's body carries risk too.

Risk accompanies anything significant. Adoption has risks,
no question about that. But when adoption is approached
with wise counsel, prayer, homework, and patience, the risks
can be greatly minimized.

### Will an adopted child feel like my child?

Yes, absolutely. It doesn't take an umbilical cord to make a
child your own. The connection is one that comes as naturally
as loving a birth child. I remember feeling light-headed the
moment tiny Ryan was placed in my arms. Time slowed to a
crawl and those moments took on a soft-focus appearance. It
was incredible beyond my expectations. He was a 26-week
preemie and was finally out of the hospital at almost four
months of age and finally weighing five pounds. When I held
him for the first time, it was just like holding a newborn.

Couples who have adopted describe the moment of having the child placed in their arms in terms that rival any birth experience (well, minus the physical pain).

*It was as emotional as if I had given birth to him. The biological mom's birthing coach and I were the only nonmedical people in the room during delivery. After Alex was born, I pushed his bassinet down the hall to the nursery, and I cried all the way. Finally, I was a mother!*                                                    —*Joy*

*When Sean was first placed in my arms in the delivery room, I was overwhelmed by the miracle of birth, overwhelmed that God would trust the protection, nurturing, and upbringing of this innocent baby to us, and overwhelmed that this birth mom selected Bob and me to raise him. I was anxious to spend my first private moments with him.*                                                  —*Paula*

Most couples feel an instant connection with their adopted child. When a child enters your life after months and years of prayer and anticipation, whether that child is birthed or adopted, the exuberance and thrill is the same. God has finally answered! All the love you've been saving for a child has finally found an outlet in this incredible human being with the face of a tiny angel.

Many couples find it divinely ironic that God places children in their lives who actually look like one adoptive parent. Does it matter that adoptive parents sometimes end up with children who look like themselves? No, but it makes the story even more interesting—and it's a reassurance that God was weaving together this family even before all the participative adults (biological and adoptive parents) were aware of what the future held.

My son and I just happen to have the same color hair, the same chin, nose, and facial shape. Everywhere we go, strangers comment on how much we favor each other: "He looks just like you." I must admit, I like to surprise them with the news that Ryan is adopted, and then credit God with putting our family together.

On the flip side, parents who adopt children with differing ethnicities enjoy the unique blend their family has. They take pleasure in their child's nationality. The fact that their child doesn't look like them doesn't matter. They are a family bound together by love, woven by the hand of God.

*Because Thomas is Russian, he looks like he could be our birth child. But with Olivia, I am asked often if she is adopted and from where (Kazakhstan). We want our children to know where they are from and to be proud of their heritage. Thomas is now three, and when asked where he is from he will say "Russia," and sometimes point it out on a map.*
— *Katie*

*Our family is made up of three nationalities—American, Nepalese, and Cambodian. We live in yet a fourth culture (Asia). When people look at me, they look down with a smile at the stroller, expecting to see cute, blonde, foreign kids. As soon as they see my children's nationalities, they look back up at me. Then they look at my husband, back at me, and back at the kids. This pattern is almost predictable! I am very proud of our children's ethnicities, but I don't even "see" their differing nationalities now. All I can see is my kids.*

*Our children are from remote villages in faraway countries. It's probable that they would have never heard the good news of Christ. We believe God reached down and plucked them from death and gave them life and the opportunity to know Him.*
— *Sherri*

## What about genetic issues?

Some couples struggle with not having a biological connection to their child. For them, an intangible comfort exists in knowing their child shares their genetic codes. They have a strong desire to pass along the family heritage via birth. Your family tree may not have adopted children anywhere on it. Maybe you fear the child won't be accepted by your parents, your aunts or uncles, your grandparents.

*When we adopted Mark he was twelve days old, and it was a first for our extended family. My husband's father had said an adopted child would never be considered his grandchild, but he turned out to be the silliest of all. We arrived at his home about 6:30 P.M. to introduce him to Mark, and by 8:00 he had called all his other children, including one in Ohio. Both sides of the family were thrilled for us and so happy to have a little baby boy added to the family.* — *Ellen*

Only you can assess your extended family's opinions on adoption, but the real issue is determining what's right for you and your spouse. If you don't adopt because of family pressure, do you want to spend the rest of your life knowing you appeased your extended family by not adopting, while you ached for the opportunity to love a child—a child you could have adopted? Carefully talk through this issue with your spouse.

*Everyone was very excited and supportive of our upcoming adoption, except for Jeff's grandmother. Jeff is the last male in his family line, and she thought we should keep trying to get pregnant. When he finally said, "This is what we are doing," she came around, and has been the best great-grandma we could have hoped for.*    —Joy

Medically speaking, having a genetic connection is handy because you know more about your own medical history than you'll know about that of an adopted child, although adoptive parents today have a chance to know a great deal more about their child's medical history than those in decades past. Birth parents often complete a medical history to pass along to adoptive parents. But don't let the need for medical predictions dissuade you from adopting. When you think about the multitudes of medical maladies on record, the chances that your birth child will develop something unforeseen are as great as those of your adopted child.

I'm thinking of two college friends who married and had two children. Both children inherited a genetic syndrome, a disease that drastically affects their day-to-day life and their life expectancy. No one in either family tree had developed the disease. No one could have predicted that the combination of these two genetic codes would produce this problem in their children. So, if you think bearing your own children is always safer than adopting, think again. Until all the ramifications of the genetic map are established, you really cannot predict exactly what you are passing on to your genetic offspring. Plus, you cannot safeguard every aspect of a pregnancy. Nothing is entirely safe. Nothing is entirely risk free.

I watched another couple turn down an adoption because the child had Down syndrome. To this day, I go back and forth between disbelief that they rejected the child and trying to respect their feelings that they weren't able to handle the situation. But they'll never know what God might have wanted to do with them and *through* them if they had taken that baby into their home.

For some reason, the factor of choice in adoption makes some people think they deserve a perfect child, though they never would hold up the same standard for the birth child they so want. If you birth a child with a defect, you wouldn't even contemplate giving up that child. You'd take him home, love him, get medical intervention as necessary, and commit to being the best parents possible for your child. Why should it be any different with an adopted child?

Is there a point where you can say it's not about you *getting* something, but it's about you *giving* what God has blessed you with—giving it to an adopted child? By stopping an adoption because the child isn't perfect, you've stopped too soon. You've not allowed yourself the opportunity for God to show you just how equipped you are (or will be) to fulfill the role of parenting this specific child.

My husband and I know from experience that you never know what you're capable of until God places you directly in circumstances that seem beyond your ability to cope. Ryan's genetic syndrome affects his walking and his joint flexibility, and his profound deafness makes us dependent on sign language, which we'll be learning the rest of our lives. But now I'm so thankful that Ryan's special needs hadn't been diagnosed when we adopted him. We probably would have been too scared to take on his medical issues. And we would have missed the biggest blessing of our lives! We never imagined we could rise to the call of parenting a special needs child; but amazingly, we are doing it day by day, and our lives are filled with laughter and joy. We have never regretted our decision for even one fraction of a moment. We are part of something bigger than us.

Maybe it comes down to deciding you're going to love whatever child God puts in your life, regardless. You could birth a child with special needs and you'd love her, regardless. Or you could work with a birth mother, learn the baby will have special needs, and embrace the opportunity. By the way, God was the first to say He would love us, regardless: "God demonstrates his own love for us in this: While we were still sinners, Christ died for us" (Rom. 5:8).

### What about the great unknown?

*Anne of Green Gables,* one of my favorite book series, tells of an orphan who goes to live on Prince Edward Island in the late 1800s when she is adopted by Murilla and Matthew Cuthbert, an aging sister and brother. They receive dire warnings from their nosy neighbor, Rachel Lind, about adopted children. She's heard stories about an adopted child who set fire to his family's house and another who poisoned her adopted family.

I laugh every time I see that part of the movie! Many people fear adoption today because of random stories about adoptive children who have turned out bad, who didn't bond with their adoptive family, or who commit some crime. We could each list children and youth who have been in trouble, regardless of whether they were adopted or not. In the broad scheme of events, only a fraction of such problems are attributed to adopted children. And of those problems, how many can truly be attributed to the fact that the child was adopted? Don't let this unfounded fear be a roadblock in your journey.

### When will we know we're ready to adopt?

The answer to this question differs for everyone. Each couple has to reach a point where they are ready to be parents to a child and ready to give a child a home, even if that child is not their flesh and blood. Sometimes emotional limitations put the brakes on infertility measures and steer you toward adoption. Sometimes financial limitations tell you when it's time to stop infertility treatments. (See chapter 7, "Setting Boundaries in the Valley of Infertility.")

It's not unusual for a husband and wife to arrive at the point of being ready to adopt at different times. Often, one spouse wants to explore every medical option until the door closes firmly shut, while the other wants to move ahead to adoption much sooner. Or a spouse may say, "I don't want to adopt," and really mean, "I'm not ready to move toward adoption right now." A gulf of indecision exists between "not right now" and "no, not ever." Though you may be uncomfortable, try to endure the conflicting thoughts and see-saw emotions as you make your way toward a decision. Give yourselves time, and even consider seeking a counselor to help you to work through the confusion.

*I'd heard that couples need closure on infertility before pursuing adoption. But working on the preliminary paperwork while waiting for infertility medications and procedures to work gave us a sense of accomplishment. We were experiencing so many dashed hopes, disappointments, and long waits that this was one of the few things that seemed positive and helped us move forward. The day our endocrinologist recommended that we pursue other avenues to parenthood, we began putting the finishing touches on our formal application packet.*          *—Paula*

### What about birth parents?
Many couples fear that birth parents will come back to reclaim their child in domestic (US) adoptions, now that open adoptions make communication much more frequent with both sets of parents. That fear alone makes many couples choose international adoption, where adoptions rarely involve communication with birth parents. Adoptive couples crave a feeling of safety that no one can ever have any possible claim to their child.

In reality, only one-tenth of 1 percent of adoptions are contested. Eighty percent stay intact until legalization, and more than 98 percent are never terminated. When an adoption is handled intelligently and by the book, there are no loopholes for birth parents who might change their minds and want their child back.

"Agencies work with lawyers in obtaining the proper relinquishments, affidavits, and waivers necessary to fulfill the law for that state," says Vicky Payne, executive director of Inheritance Adoptions in Wichita Falls, Texas. "The agency is more likely to be able to determine in advance whether or not the birth parent plans to follow through with an adoption plan. An agency will have other parents who have placed for adoption who share their experiences with the expectant mother and father."

**Adoption lawyer or adoption agency?**

Obviously, adopting a child isn't as easy as transferring the title of a car from one owner to the other. Both are legal transactions, but adoption is universally more complex. If you think it's simply about finding a birth mother who wants to give you her child and then filing some paperwork in court to make it official, then you're in for some legal surprises.

When couples definitely decide to adopt, they must choose whether to affiliate with an adoption agency that will handle their adoption throughout the entire process or hire an adoption lawyer to process legal paperwork once an adoptable child is located.

If you decide to explore using an adoption lawyer, do your homework. Don't just grab a name out of the phone book. Ask friends and family for names of adoption lawyers in your city or state who have done a good job. Call and ask about fees, processes, and legal requirements. Does the lawyer know of any birth mothers currently trying to find adoptive parents? Ask about the adoption laws in your state. What is the waiting period between placement and final adoption? Ask what lengths the lawyer will go to in order to obtain parental rights' releases from the birth mother and all possible birth fathers.

While most adoption lawyers are completely adequate, I believe a couple may be nurtured and helped along in the process far more by an adoption agency. The agency has the welfare of both parties in mind—the adoptive parents and the birth parents. The agency is your intermediary in dealing with the birth mother, which can be an emotional lifesaver when you've been through the wringer with years of infertility treatments. You'll save yourself even more duress by letting the agency be your go-between, your advocate in dealing with birth parents and adoption proceedings.

Here are six tips for choosing an agency:

*1. Ask adoptive parents for opinions about the agency they used.* You're looking for an agency that has a good record of being an advocate for adoptive parents, keeping them informed along the way, offering advice about what to do next, and more. Warning: Don't affiliate with an adoption agency that operates primarily through the Internet. Anyone can hawk anything on the Web—babies included.

**2. Begin by considering which adoption agency seems to match your needs and your financial boundaries.** Call several agencies for general information about their adoption policies. Ask to receive any printed materials that overview the agency's adoption procedures (a nominal charge may be required for information packets).

**3. Read the agencies' information to get a feel for their processes.** Ask your agency how many children they place each year, how many adoptions are finalized each year, and exactly what the adoption fee covers (and doesn't cover). Some agencies find a birth mother for you; others train you to locate a birth mother through ads. Most ask you to rally friends and relatives to join you in looking for a birth mother who might be interested in placing her child for adoption. These efforts to involve adoptive parents in finding a birth mother are because more birth mothers are keeping their babies, free of the social stigma that unwed pregnancy had in years past. Therefore, it takes more manpower to find adoptable children. The flip side of this involvement is that parents generally wait much less time for a baby. Whereas hopeful parents in other decades were told to expect a wait of many years (one couple was told to expect to wait nine years), today's adoptive parents sometimes are matched within weeks, months, or a year or two. Few wait longer than that.

**4. Determine what financial resources are available for adoption expenses.** Remember that the bulk of your expenses will be related to the adoption agency fee. Additional expenses may be required for the birth mother's delivery or prenatal care, court costs, home study costs, travel/lodging to another state (if the birth mother lives elsewhere). Investigate whether your health insurance company will pay for a birth mother's hospital stay if the child is to be adopted by you.

**5. After you've narrowed the field of agencies that interest you, attend the information session the agencies offer.**

Attending these sessions won't commit you to choose a particular agency. It is just one step you take in the decision-making process.

**6. *Determine which agency is the best fit for you.*** Move forward with interviews, filling out forms and biographical information, paying adoption fees, etc.

After the home study is completed, your forms are filled out, and your biographical information is on file with your agency, you wait and pray and prepare for how God is going to move in your lives as He brings you in contact with a birth mother.

### What do adopted children think about their birth parents and adopted parents?

Here are three very different perspectives from three adults who were adopted as babies. Paula, Ray, and Lane's adoptions were all closed, which was the only option at the time.

Paula, the second child adopted by her parents (Ellen and Paul), has wondered about her birth mother "for as long as I can remember." What did she look like? Who was she? Why did she give her up for adoption? At age eighteen, Paula began formally looking for her birth mother, but with no results. At twenty-four she moved to Austin, Texas, and learned her birth records were on file there and that she could list her name in a registry to match birth parents and adopted children. Eight years later she got a call from the registry with news that her birth father had registered. This was the registry's first match and they didn't quite know what to do! Soon she met her father and her younger sister. He helped her locate her birth mother, who had three sons.

*I don't remember ever fantasizing that my birth family was better; I only remember being curious about them. I've always felt support from my adoptive mother to find my birth family. She is my mom, and there is no other. The bond you have with your adopted family cannot be broken. My father and brother died while I was in my twenties, so it became increasingly important for me to know if I had any biological siblings who wanted to meet me. Now, the newness of locating each other has worn off, and we are all just families like anyone else. We email, send cards and gifts, and try to get together whenever possible.*

Ray came to his parents through the referral of a family physician who knew of an unplanned pregnancy in the next town. After adopting Ray, his adoptive parents later adopted a baby girl. "My parents told me from the beginning that I was adopted," Ray said. "They used to tell the story of me as a toddler saying to people, 'I am special. I am adopted.' When I was about ten, I asked my father what it meant to be adopted. He carefully explained it to me, and it didn't seem to be a big deal to me."

He never wanted to meet his birth parents; and even when his parents discovered his birth grandmother, he still wasn't interested in meeting her. "My younger sister, however, wondered a lot about her birth parents, especially during her teen years. Our feelings were very different even though we were brought up in the same environment."

After Ray and his wife, Janis, had their second son, concerns arose about his motor development; an MRI showed extra fluid in one area of the baby's brain. "I wondered if there was any medical history I needed to be aware of. My mother helped me locate my birth mother through a birth aunt. And I learned that my birth father died soon after I was born."

Ray found out there were no known neurological problems in the family, but his birth mother didn't want to talk to him directly. "I was disappointed and felt rejected a second time. I wanted to share how God had richly blessed my life. In some way, I wanted my birth mother to be proud and to feel she had made the right decision."

Lane grew up as the only child of an adoptive couple. "They were the best parents I could ever have hoped to have," he said. "They were my real parents in every sense of the word." Although he grew up knowing he was adopted, his parents didn't focus on the day he was placed with them, as many parents do today. (It's often called "Gotcha Day.") "My adoption wasn't something we talked about, so it wasn't something I thought about very often. Sometime in college, it dawned on me in a conscious way that I was adopted." His extended family respected his parents' wishes by not discussing Lane's adoption. "I think some of my first cousins still don't know I was adopted."

Lane and his wife, Deana, who have had infertility problems of their own, are now parents to two children, Taylor and Avery. Lane has never had the desire to locate his biological parents, even though his parents died by the time he was thirty-one. "The only thing I'd like to know from my biological parents is some medical history," he said, "and that's for the sake of my children. Some people might think I have some gaps to fill in my life now that my parents have passed away. But no one can take the place of my parents."

Today's domestic adoptions are more likely to be open or semiopen, meaning that children can grow up with knowledge or even interaction with their birth parent(s). (International adoptions are closed, offering little or no opportunity to know anything at all about the birth parents.) Of the many adoptive families I know personally, only one has a relationship with the birth family which is a little tense and a little overinvolved. All the others have settled into a comfortable pattern of contact periodically via pictures, letters, and occasional phone calls. Their children are secure and well-adjusted within loving families.

## My confession

I'll be honest with you: I've always wanted to adopt a child. Not everyone feels that way, but I've wanted to adopt for as long as I can remember. From an early age, I realized there was a part of my heart that would one day want to embrace a child I hadn't birthed. Why? I couldn't help but think about my own upbringing—a warm, secure family with parents who loved me unconditionally, helped me reach my goals, and gave me deep roots for life and faith. I wanted to give that security to a child who hadn't been born into it. Sure, someone else *might* do it, someone else *could* do it, but I knew I was *capable* of doing it, so why shouldn't I step up to the plate myself?

Fortunately, my husband felt the same way. Edward surprised me while we were dating when he told me he'd always wanted to adopt too. We later agreed on an ideal plan to birth a few of our own, then adopt. Well, the ideal didn't pan out, so we moved on. For us, building our family through adoption was simply *another* option, not a *lesser* option.

Have you really laid your fears and concerns about adoption before the Lord? My prayer is that God has allayed some of your worries and, whether or not you go on to adopt, that you will be able to see adoption from a more truthful (and dare I say *miraculous?*) perspective.

## Moses, a cross-cultural adoption

Jochebed watched her friends' babies die at Pharaoh's command to throw all Hebrew boys in the Nile River. Probably a little scared but fiercely determined, Jochebed got creative when she could hide her infant son no longer. At three months of age, she whipped up a waterproof basket to float her baby along the Nile's reeds. Pharaoh's daughter was bathing in the Nile and saw the basket, discovered the baby, and decided to make him her own (Exod. 1–2).

Ever wonder what Jochebed's long-term plan was? I sure have. Was she planning for someone in Pharaoh's household to find her son and have mercy on him? (Talk about wishful thinking!) Was the basket simply a stopgap measure until she could think of some other way to hide him? Did she plan to hide him in increasingly larger baskets until she could somehow sneak him back into the Hebrew population without arousing suspicion from the Egyptian overseers? Maybe she was trying to split hairs: "Well, sir, my son *is* in the Nile River, so I've fulfilled the edict. He's just not *dead* in the Nile."

We'll never know Jochebed's plan, nor will we know what Jochebed named her baby. The name Moses, first mentioned in

Exodus 2:10, came from Pharaoh's daughter. But we do know the results of her plan: Moses was nursed by Jochebed, raised in an adoptive home (just the local palace down the road), and eventually became the unparalleled leader of the Hebrews. Like his Hebrew biological mother, Moses was a little scared but fiercely determined. And like his Egyptian adoptive mother, he was inclined to see the people's needs and have mercy on them. These women never imagined they were forging such a momentous adoption across cultures, which would eventually separate the two cultures forever.

# Chapter 11

# Sitting on the Fence:
## Choosing between Parenthood and Child-free Living

*I watch my youth slipping away. I watch my childbearing years evaporate, empty and silent. I wonder if I'm supposed to have kids to carry on the banner of Christ. I wonder if I want kids, with the polarities they bring — incredible joy and inexplicable pain, hope and devastation, potential and disappointment. The risks are high; the outcome is unknown with each child. Such unpredictable results. Yesterday I admitted to myself that I didn't want kids . . . .at least at that moment. I just can't decide, and I don't think Edward can, either. I asked him point-blank last night, and he fumbled around until he finally said, "I guess so." Why are we so stupidly indecisive on this? Others seem to know one way or the other. We just vacillate.* —*my journal, June 15, 1995*

I wore the paint off the spot on the proverbial fence where I sat for several years. I'd look to one side and see the fields of parenthood—colorful, busy, full of families. Then there was the other side, the rolling hills where couples choose to live without children of their own, filling their lives with meaning and purpose in a variety of ways. Couples who just find themselves pregnant can't understand the struggle, because the decision is taken out of their hands when she turns up pregnant. No one, in fact, understands unless they've sat on that fence themselves. But infertile couples can spend a lot of time trying to determine whether parenthood is God's plan for our lives. Some of you already know parenthood is what you want—no question about it. But for a great many of us, the fact that we're working so hard to get pregnant gives us time to question just how far we should push our efforts, just how long we should beat our heads against the wall before we stop trying to bear a child or adopt.

Choosing to remain childless is an option for any couple. But it's important to make the distinction: Childlessness as a *lifestyle* is different from childlessness as a *predicament*. Having no children is as much a lifestyle choice as is the decision to become parents. On the flip side, childlessness as a *predicament* is what we spend effort and money trying to change.

In thinking about childlessness as a lifestyle, a better term is needed, one that's not weighted down with so much need for interpretation: *Child-free living* is a more affirming way to describe couples with no children. Some couples choose child-free living before they even know they're infertile. They just never want to have children. But what about couples who have engaged the Big-I monster and then opt for a child-free life? How do they come to that decision, since their first intent was to be parents? How do they make the emotional transition from childlessness to a child-free mentality? Still others find themselves relegated to childlessness after years of not getting pregnant, never making the crossover from the remorse of childlessness to the sense of peace that can come from choosing to be child-free.

It's a big fence and a lot of people have sat on it through the years. Here are a few of their stories.

### Karen and Peter: A change of plans
Before she'd even met Peter, Karen had mapped out her life. "I had a life plan, and marriage and children were not an accessory I'd considered. My career was my priority. And my life plan was going according to schedule. But things changed when I met Peter in the air force." It was one of those rare, love-at-first-sight romances; and when they started dating, Karen watched her life plan change. They married in 1988, and "that's when we first started discussing the family issue. We decided that, yes, we were interested in having a family."

A move to Michigan brought more to Karen's life than just a change of geography, though. "I discovered something interesting about Peter. I knew that his sister was a Christian artist, but Peter never discussed church and never attended. Well, when we moved, Peter jumped back into church life full swing. That left me in a bit of shock, since I didn't grow up in a Christian household and had never been to church. I started attending with him, and after lots of prayers and patience from friends who answered my endless questions, I finally became a Christian after two years.

"Incredibly, two months after accepting Christ I became pregnant! I thought, 'This Christian thing is great. Now God is getting to the blessing by allowing me to be pregnant.'"

But Karen miscarried, and then a year later she had a second miscarriage. Infertility testing and drugs, depression, and marital strain followed the initial grief of the first miscarriage. Karen and Peter went to a marriage counselor and Karen also got counseling to help her work through the grief related to losing two babies to miscarriage.

"Peter really slowed me down and made me think about why we were having children. I had never really been challenged by anything that I couldn't defeat. I'd been brought up with the concept that if you work hard enough, then you can get it done. I took that approach to getting pregnant. I am not a quitter, and it was hard for me to face that when it got down to it, neither Peter nor I felt 'compelled' to have our own children. Once I did, we stopped the medical experiments."

A call from a woman at church instigated a change in Karen's life. The woman knew about a job opening at a local university for an academic advisor. "In hindsight, I realize that was definitely a 'God thing.' The job was a perfect fit, and it allowed me to slowly get my legs back under me."

Karen began to see that God was using all her past experiences in this new job, and now she feels "complete." "Somewhere I read that the true measure of becoming a Christian is to accept the dreams that Christ has for your life instead of insisting on your own dreams. It's still easy for me to wander back into trying to make a plan of my own."

Karen hasn't chosen a lesser route by not becoming a parent. She has submitted her own dreams before God and is embracing the opportunities He is giving her. Karen and Peter believe they are fulfilling their roles in the Great Commission, just as He planned for them to do.

**Roy and Dirce: Finding their self-worth from God alone**
In another part of the world, a couple from America tried to
have children, but later made the choice to be child-free. Roy
and Dirce have been missionaries since 1990, serving first in
Costa Rica and now in Mexico. Roy works in theological education, and Dirce ministers through outreach evangelism.

Roy and Dirce intended to have children, wanted children,
expected children. "We made it a matter of prayer together,"
Roy said, "and we both were very excited about the prospect
of having children together."

During their first furlough in 1995, they went to several
specialists to try to assess why they weren't getting pregnant.
They even attempted one IVF, but it wasn't successful. "We're
still not sure of all the reasons why we haven't been able to
have children," Roy says.

Roy and Dirce have some remarkable things to say about
how they found peace with a lifestyle that hasn't included
children of their own:

*We've gone through sad times because of not being able to have chil-
dren, but we've learned that our ultimate worth doesn't come from
how many children we have; it comes from God alone.*

*We remember that God is worthy of our trust. We believe that
God is love—He would never withhold anything from us that would
be for the good of the kingdom. God is wise—He knows what is best
for us and the ministry He has entrusted to us. God is all-powerful.
He chose to perform a miracle in giving Abraham and Sarah a child
in their old age, so we have no doubt that He can do it. Therefore we
trust Him.*

**Cheryl and David: Infertility confirmed their decision**
While they were dating, Cheryl and David discovered that
neither one of them felt particularly drawn to having children.
"We talked about the fact that we didn't want to have children," Cheryl said. "We both devoted so much time to our
careers, which we enjoyed. We put it in God's hands and
believed that He had brought us together, preparing us both
for a life that didn't include children of our own."

They had only been married a year when Cheryl was diagnosed with endometriosis. Several surgeries followed, but a

hysterectomy at age twenty-eight finally gave her relief from the painful condition. "The many surgical procedures just reinforced our decision that we were not supposed to have children," she said. "But we had to convince my doctor that we had given extensive thought to adoption if we should change our minds and want to start a family."

They heard a lot of "Well, you can always adopt." "These comments basically ignored the fact that before being unable to conceive, we had made a decision to be childless," Cheryl says.

What everyone wants (and needs), whether they choose to have kids or not, is *peace* with their decision. *Your life* is a gift God has given you. Coming to terms with the lifestyle you choose is important in order to embrace your life in a healthy, fulfilling way. Children can be additional gifts to your life, but they shouldn't be your only key to happiness.

"Peace with our decision has always remained a constant," Cheryl says. "However, I can't say that I haven't wondered what motherhood must be like."

That's a fair observation. Wondering about motherhood and pining away for it are entirely different. Cheryl and David live active, fulfilled, child-free lives. "God brought us together, and He keeps us together with love and joy for each other."

## Helen: A late-bloomer

Helen is in her eighties, so her years of infertility are far behind her, but her story is characteristic of the infertile women in her era. She didn't have many options open when pregnancy didn't "just happen" in the 1940s as she and her husband Robert began trying to have a family.

*Our money was scarce and I didn't know much about infertility and medical helps. There weren't a lot of options at that time. One month my period was late. I thought I was pregnant, and Robert was so excited. But I wasn't pregnant after all, and we were both so disappointed. I thought God didn't see fit to give us children.*

*Robert loved children very much. I remember coming home from work more than once to find him sitting on the grass telling stories to several neighbors' children.*

*I envied my friends who were having children. We felt very much left out and didn't get invited to events sometimes, and I felt it was because we had no children. We wrote to some adoption agencies, but because of our ages, we could only get much older children. We felt we had to accept the fact that childlessness was God's will.*

*Not having children was one of the greatest regrets of my life. It still saddens me.*

After 42 years of "a happy, wonderful marriage," Robert died. Eventually, Helen began attending a grief support group, and it was there that she met Henry. They married in 1988. Henry and his first wife (deceased) had had a large family, so Helen "inherited" five married children, fifteen grandchildren, and six great-grandchildren.

*His children are all very sweet to me. I love them all. When his daughter came to see us early in our marriage, she said, "Dad, you're in good hands." Another daughter said, "My dad knows how to pick his women." His son sent me a basket of flowers on Mother's Day, with a card that said, "Thank you for loving Dad and taking care of him." A few years ago I was standing in the hallway with one son, looking at all the pictures of kids and grandkids. I said, "I wish I'd had kids to give Henry some competition." His son replied, "Helen, we are your kids." I thought that was so sweet. I guess I was a late bloomer as a mother, thank the Lord.*

### Ethel and Haskell: Content with family and friends

Like Helen and Robert, Ethel and Haskell were married in the 1940s, a time noted for its limited help for infertile couples. "A short while after we married, I realized there was a problem, so I went to the doctor," Ethel said. "I knew very little about infertility."

The doctor discussed adoption with Ethel, and after a while Ethel decided to talk to her husband about it. "Haskell wouldn't consent to an adoption. I was disappointed, but I loved Haskell so much that I didn't get a complex about it."

Ethel filled her life with her activities at church, helping Haskell with the real estate business and caring for family members—her mother-in-law, two uncles who had no children, and her sister who lived with her for four years. Her nieces, nephews, and friends' children have been recipients of her love and generosity through the decades.

*They're wonderful, and I've been very close to them. For Haskell and me, our dreams were to be with each other and do what we could for our family. As busy as my life has been, I don't think I'd want to change anything. I thank God for the joys I've had through the years with my family and friends.*

## A little advice

As with any long-lasting, life-altering decision, you have to think about your motives in choosing whether or not to have children. Roy and Dirce gave serious thought to whether or not they should choose child-free living or pursue nonbirth options such as adoption or foster parenting.

"I would encourage anyone who is thinking about not having children to consider and evaluate your motives," Roy said. "Some couples don't have children for selfish reasons: they don't want the bother or 'danger' of children, or they don't want children to get in the way of their career." On the flip side, some people *have* children for selfish reasons: to feel wanted, to feel loved, to live out their dreams through their kids, or to fit in with society.

All couples should consider the four topics below as they assess their decision to be parents or to remain child-free.

*1. Consider this time without children as a unique part of your life.* From my perspective on the just-shy side of forty, those twenty-something years brought life phases tumbling one after another. College, job, marriage, and children were prescribed rites of passage, and it seemed we couldn't really consider ourselves complete until we'd accomplished them all. We get in such a rush to settle down and accumulate all the trappings of what makes life acceptable in our culture.

But for the couple who is waiting (by choice or by circumstances) to have children, or for the single adult who waits to marry, life shouldn't be viewed as empty, but as full of opportunity. You've been given the gift of time. For the most part, your time is your own, so your interests and ministry goals can be pursued at will. You can go do missions for a week, a month, or a year or two. You can change your life direction. You can give Christ's love to people who will never cross your paths once you're responsible for the health, safety, and growth of children.

You have much love to give, and parenthood isn't the only outlet for it. Think outside the box. Ask God if there's something incredible you should be doing with your life right now as you wait for children or try to decide whether parenthood is for you.

*2. Explore your sense of call (i.e., your dream, your goal) to parenthood or to being child-free.* I sat in a doctor's office not long after our questions about infertility started to crop up. The doctor looked me straight in the eye and said, "Are you pursuing parenthood because you really feel you should raise children, or is it because you feel pressured to?" He went on to explain how family members can push a couple into feeling obligated to have children, or even how our culture has unspoken expectations that every couple will eventually have or acquire offspring. He gave me a glimpse into his own life when he said he "probably shouldn't have been a father." He thoroughly enjoyed his career, his practice, and interacting with patients, so much so that his family life suffered.

People who fall into parenthood without a sense of calling can become frustrated, resentful, and impatient with the never-ending demands that children make on their lives and lifestyles. In all honesty, even those who enter parenthood intentionally and with a sense of divine calling feel the same way at times. For some couples, the vocation, job, volunteer work, or ministry that God has brought to them is enough of a lifework in and of itself. Others can honestly testify that they've just never had an interest in raising children. It doesn't mean they don't enjoy and love children—they just don't want to raise their own. It's a decision that should be made carefully and consciously.

*3. Don't be saddled by the fear that you need children to care for you in your old age.* Children can do that, but you have no guarantee that they will. No one knows if their children will be emotionally or physically able to support an elderly parent.

And no one knows for sure that their children will outlive them.

Today's childless adults (and even single adults) are not in the same predicament as in years past. Most adults have retirement plans, annuities, and pensions to provide monetarily for their later years. Women can work for their own livelihood. Children should be wanted, birthed, and adopted for higher reasons—not as the means to a secure end. Children are not an "old-age insurance policy."

**4. If you decide to remain childless, embrace the wholeness of being child-free.** Once you have determined you've had all the fertility treatments you can afford (or endure), and that adoption and fostering aren't for you, then determine to see yourself not as a childless couple, but as a child-free couple. It's more than semantics. It's a matter of perspective. Choose to see yourself as fulfilled exactly as you are.

If you and your spouse find yourselves more and more comfortable with the decision to be child-free, make plans to mark the decision with some degree of ceremony. Consider a time of prayer and thanksgiving to God for bringing you to a sense of peace about this decision. Write in your journal the thoughts and events that led you to this choice so you'll have a permanent record of the chronology of the decision-making process. Commemorate your decision by investing in the future: make a donation to a favorite charity, pledge a monthly contribution to help children in a needy country, plant trees at a children's home. Let this mark the beginning of how you will look for ways to pass along the legacy of love that God has given you.

# Chapter 12

# Learning to Trust God through Infertility

*There was a time when we both wondered what we had done to deserve this. God had answered our prayers by bringing us together, so where was He now? Jeff was able to pray through it more than I could. I wanted to know where God had gone, and why He wasn't allowing me to get pregnant!*

*—Joy*

We inadvertently think that a close walk with God will give us some assurance of getting out of life the major things we hope for: health; a happy marriage; healthy children; and at least the basics in food, water, and shelter. When a major foe enters the picture—cancer, job loss, or infertility—it doesn't take long for us to judge our experiences as unjust and unfair.

We conveniently forget that this God from whom we're demanding our version of fair play is also the God who chooses not to condemn us to eternal death. This is the same God who provided redemption through His Son, Jesus Christ. This is the God who pardons us when we confess our sin and accept His path of forgiveness and restoration.

But we don't just say, "Oh, life isn't fair. Thanks for the information." We can't just get on with life even though we acknowledge that truth. The spiritual implications of infertility put deep gouges in our faith. We feel anger toward the God we love. That anger makes us question our faith—is it wrong to be angry at God? Am I doing something that keeps Him from answering me? Why would a God of love let me experience this? We feel God has double-crossed us, even betrayed us by not giving us children, especially when we've made it perfectly clear that we want to raise them to love and honor the Lord. And in the midst of struggling with negotiating the whys, we have to figure out how to maintain our walk with God, or if we even want to. We know we *should* hang on to God during this trial, but we find ourselves less than anxious to pray and meditate on His Word when all we can think of is that we're really ticked off with our Creator.

### "I don't understand, God" versus "I don't understand God"

The comma changes the meaning of the sentence, but both statements are common cries in infertility. We don't understand why God allows these horrible things to happen to us, and we discover that we just don't understand God like we thought we did.

The intersection between our faith and our quest for parenthood is fraught with questions, many of them "if . . . then" questions:

- *If God loves me, then why isn't He giving us a child?*
- *If I'm a believer, then why isn't God answering my prayer?*
- *If we're committed to raising a child in a godly home, then why can't we have a child as easily as those Hollywood stars who just live together?*
- *If I'm doing my part as a Christian, then why isn't God doing His part as Provider?*

What have your questions been? What questions would you add? Jot them in the margin.

These questions fall into the category of I Don't Understand God's Ways. No kidding. We don't understand why God gives babies to unmarried movie stars, to child abusers, and to people who won't give a child a stable, loving home. Just this week in our city, a well-to-do CPA shot his two daughters, aged six and nine, in the head, because he wanted to permanently hurt his ex-wife. Why did God allow a man like that to be a parent?

Instead of chasing that rabbit, let's move to the bigger issue: Why does God let bad things (like infertility) happen to good people (like Christians)? This question leads us to others:

Why do so many bad people have rampant fertility? Why does pain afflict those who choose righteousness, who try valiantly to live according to God's Word?

We don't understand why God doesn't readily answer the prayers of decent, God-fearing, infertile people. But God never promised us that in our earthly understanding and limitations, we would be able to comprehend His ways. Instead, He says the opposite: "'For my thoughts are not your thoughts, neither are your ways my ways,' declares the Lord. 'As the heavens are higher than the earth, so are my ways higher than your ways and my thoughts than your thoughts'" (Isa. 55:8–9 NIV).

Bridget's baby died of Sudden Infant Death Syndrome. Meg's children drowned in a boating accident. Elizabeth's long-awaited baby died at birth. Many of you reading this book have already lost a baby, yet you still have to fight infertility for the privilege and risk of bearing another. These unanswerables grip our hearts with grief. No, we cannot understand why God allows such horrible losses. In this life, we simply will *never* have the comprehension to understand completely. So where do we go from here?

## Learning to live without understanding

Many Christians can't bear to live without understanding why they're being subjected to tragedy. They look and look for reasons:

- *Did someone come to know Christ because of my pain?*
- *Did I experience personal spiritual renewal because of walking through this valley?*
- *Did someone return to their walk with God after seeing what we've been through?*
- *Have I become more equipped to comfort others because of my experience?*

Trying to find the reason *why* is really just searching for a spiritual/psychological bandage to stick on your heart and mind. Seeing that God brought something good out of our pain will (we hope) help us to balance those scales of eternal justice. "Oh, so *that's* why God allowed it."

You've probably heard, "In time, you'll understand why this had to happen; not now, but later God will show you." Nice try, but the truth is, we won't always get a glimpse of the why behind the tragedy. What really rubs me the wrong way is the phrase, "why this had to happen." These words only undermine a person's right to grieve openly and completely. It robs a person of her right to feel pain because it suggests that the loss will be justified by the eventual gain.

My husband returned stunned from the recent funeral of a co-worker in his late forties who died unexpectedly in his sleep. His wife and two young children faced the worst experience of their lives; yet at the service, the priest told them that they were *blessed* because their husband/father had died. *Blessed!* He specifically told the little boy, about age eleven, that he was blessed that his father was gone because God would use that tragedy to mold his character for the future. Then he mentioned a notable religious figure whose mother died when her son was about the same age, explaining that her death made him what he is today. My husband and his co-workers wondered what the bereaved family thought about the funeral. To them, it wasn't very comforting.

If we study a crisis long and hard enough, we can usually squeeze out *some* reason why this grief and pain "had to" afflict us. But instead of grasping for the rationale behind why God let it happen, I suggest we move toward acknowledging that God's ways are beyond our understanding. This humbles us before our heavenly Father. It doesn't mean we're negating or suppressing our grief, but we're coming to terms with our lack of understanding. I would personally rather come to terms with living with the unknown than try to justify such losses. It seems more honest to say, "I don't know why, and I'll never know why, at least not while I'm on this earth."

Does God bring good things out of bad? Of course. But does He inflict bad things on us so He can turn around and sprout good results? I'm not convinced He works this way.

### So how does God work?
We live in a world that is subject to imperfections, and our faith doesn't make us immune to experiencing those imperfections. Infertility is one of those imperfections.

Mankind lost its perfected state when sin entered via the world's first parents, Adam and Eve. God is allowing sin and its consequences to reign on earth for a while. Even though as believers we are forgiven of our sins, we are still subject to the consequences of this imperfect, fallen world. The imperfections we encounter mean there are pitfalls and dangers, and we Christians can trip and fall just as easily as the next guy. We bear the consequences of living in this world, some of which have caused our infertility problems, some of which have caused our miscarriages.

A friend lost her mother when a beloved doctor's hand slipped during a procedure, puncturing her lung irreparably. The doctor isn't perfect, and even though his intentions were good, he made a mistake. There was no oversight or malice on his part, and the family doesn't hold it against him. But a dearly loved woman died. Have some good things come of it? Yes. But can we really say God instigated the doctor's major mistake so that minor benefits could result from the woman's death?

Being part of the human race, Christians aren't exempt from the ramifications of a world in which sin's consequences run rampant. By living in the last part of the twentieth century, our bodies have been influenced by modern medicines, illnesses, heredity, and the environment. For some reason, all of these combined to give me a whopping case of endometriosis and the inability to conceive.

But God doesn't jump in and override the natural consequences of living in this world. He doesn't divinely heal every case of sperm antibodies, save every troubled pregnancy, or open every barren womb. The Creator watches as sin's consequences play out on the history of humanity, knowing that ultimately He will step in and bring sin's stronghold to an end. (Sin is already defeated because of Christ's death on the cross, but the world awaits the final redemption at Christ's Second Coming. See Heb. 9:28.) Until then, the imperfect world we live in is full of naturally occurring mistakes.

For those who are victims of the natural consequences of this world (and this includes everyone), God offers Himself as the Comforter to those who are hurting, and He weaves together the imperfect circumstances so that some good can come from the shattered dreams of those involved. "And we know that in all things God works for the good of those who love him, who have been called according to his purpose," states the overly-quoted-in-bad-times Romans 8:28. Notice that it doesn't say that all things *are* good, but that God *works* in all things to *bring about good* for those who love Him.

God has "brought about good" if someone comes to know Christ as Savior because of your testimony after your two failed in vitro fertilizations and one miscarriage, but it doesn't mean that the loss of your babies was the required down payment for that person's eternal gain. God has worked for good when someone is helped because of your wisdom and experience after your infertility struggles, but it doesn't mean your pain was the sacrifice required for them to benefit. God sees the mess that sin and its consequences have brought to our lives and He brings something good out of the ashes by intricately interweaving lives and destinies so that the truth of His love for all humanity is made known.

### More questions that bug us

The questions we ask during trials make us dig deeper into our faith. The questions themselves are neither good nor bad, so don't berate yourself for asking the questions. (And don't let anyone else do it either.) The questions are simply reflections of your emotional and spiritual involvement in a very difficult problem. There may or may not be concrete answers out there, but you never lose when you sit down and think hard about why you believe what you've always *said* you believe. Try to dissect questions and discern what's behind them in order to figure out what this tells you about yourself and your faith journey.

### 1. Is my infertility a punishment for a past sin in my life?

Punishment, no. Consequence, maybe. Susan's abortion procedure led to a life-threatening infection that affected the viability of her reproductive organs. Infertility was a consequence of a surgical procedure. But that's not the same as punishment from God. Not even close. Another woman had a similar infection set in after an appendectomy in her preteen years. She, too, was rendered infertile. Her appendectomy and Susan's abortion are miles apart ethically, yet both experienced infertility. The consequence Susan experienced was not due to the *ethical* fact that she had an abortion, but to the *physical* fact.

*But wasn't infertility a punishment in biblical times?* A few times in the Bible, temporary infertility was doled out by God on an entire group. But in each case, it wasn't so much punishment from God as it was protection. Consider Sarah, wife of Abraham. She was to be the recipient of the post-menopausal conception and the birth of Isaac in her old age. Because of Abraham's fear of being killed by Pharaoh and later by King Abimelech of Gerar, Abraham let these two rulers take Sarah into their harems, each time telling them she was his sister (a half-truth). Apparently both Pharaoh and King Abimelech (and their households) were stricken in some way so that neither could consummate their union with Sarah. When both learned Sarah was the wife of Abraham, they immediately returned her to her husband. (Read Sarah and Abraham's story in chapter 13, "Infertile Women of the Bible.")

In Numbers 5:11–31, barrenness was a potential consequence of a divine lie detector test. God gave Moses a plan for discerning if adultery occurred by having the suspected woman drink "bitter water," which would afflict her only if she were guilty, causing her to be severely ill, to miscarry (if pregnant), and to remain barren. This wasn't poisoned water, just water with a little dirt in it and a little ink from the scroll. God knew whether adultery had occurred, and this was His way of bringing out a sin committed in secrecy. Innocent women would not be affected by the water.

The Old Testament is full of huge "if . . . then" warnings from God to His people, the Hebrews. If they obeyed Him and didn't worship false gods, then the Lord would bless them. If they strayed (a frequent problem), then they reaped a long list of consequences of their disobedience. In contrast, the New Testament offers a bright, new covenant through the birth, death, and resurrection of Jesus Christ. God initiated a new standard between Himself and His people, which now includes anyone who accepts His Son as Savior. His love and forgiveness are key themes. We have the opportunity to live under that new covenant, to know complete and total forgiveness, when we acknowledge Jesus Christ as the Son of God and the One who takes away our sin.

### 2. Is there a "broken" area of my life that I need to address?

See if any of these prayers sound familiar:

- *Lord, is there an unconfessed sin that I need to bring to You?*
- *Is there someone I need to apologize to?*
- *Are You withholding children from us just to get our attention, so we'll finally volunteer for that homeless ministry?*

When we try to dig up unconfessed sin, unresolved relationships, and areas of disobedience, we're focusing on the broken aspects of our lives. It's tempting to think that if we fix all the broken areas, then God will be happier with us and give us that baby we've been praying for. Of course, it's a good idea to look for unconfessed sin in your life, to apologize as needed, and follow the urges you get from God regarding ministry. But what is driving your desire to fix those broken areas?

Our culture's work ethic seeps into our prayer lives: Fix what's wrong and you'll be rewarded. Work hard in your job and you'll get a promotion. Work hard in your yard and you'll enjoy a beautiful lawn. Live right for God and He will give you the desires of your heart.

Whoa! David wrote in Psalm 37:4: "Delight yourself in the Lord and he will give you the desires of your heart." This is true, isn't it? Yes, but we have to ask where the desires of our heart come from. Are they earthly desires or are they truly God-centered desires, the kind that we allow Him to place in our hearts? And take a close look at the first part of that verse: "Delight yourself in the Lord." Completely, totally find your satisfaction in God. Once you've done that, the desires of your heart will be in line with His.

No doubt there have been times in your life when the desires of your heart were much more selfish than your current desire for a child. The desire for a better car or a raise in pay are in a wholly different category than the desire for a child. The deep ache for a child is noble, almost virtuous, some would say. The desire to raise a child in a godly home is certainly commendable. But one desire is as self-serving as the next if God didn't put it there to begin with.

Ask yourself, "Am I willing to stand before God and relinquish my desire for a child and my consuming desire for parenthood?" Your answer will begin to tell you whether the desire was put there by God or not. Prying our own desires out of our hearts is like trying to pull moist fingers off a frozen metal pipe—it's painful. A desire that God has authored is one that we return to Him much more easily than a desire we have authored ourselves. Lay your parental desires and longings before the Lord (repeatedly, if necessary). Then remind yourself that God definitely can be trusted with the results.

### 3. Have I done something to cause this?

If *you* do something, then *God* will be expected to respond in a predictable way. *I've been faithful in my walk with Christ since I was a child, so why isn't God answering my prayer?* This kind of thinking sets you up as the one who can control, influence, or manipulate how God acts or reacts.

I, for one, have been guilty of it. I realized I'd been praying cause-and-effect prayers when I read about a man who said he had never uttered a personal prayer in his entire life. He'd said a few rote prayers in his rare appearances in church, but he had never addressed God personally. Then one day he was standing over the hospital bed of his critically injured daughter. He found himself constructing his first personal appeal to God. From that point on, he began to pray regularly and, you guessed it, his daughter recovered.

I was just plain angry when I read that story! Not angry that his daughter had recovered, but angry that God was not answering my prayers as He had answered that man's. I've uttered "personal prayers" since I was a child! Later I realized I was expecting my past good behavior (the cause) to bring about the answered prayers (the effect) I so wanted.

Have you been praying in this way?

### 4. Where's God in all this?

When life is great, we see God's hand in everything, from little things like parking places that open up at the right moment to big things like extra money that just turns up in the checking account. But when life hits rocky terrain, we tend to overlook the handiwork because we're focusing on the bigger problems in our lives. Oh, you're still looking for His hand in your life, but it's primarily in the big prayer requests—that an IVF will work or that a new job will get you out from under financial strain. The importance of the issue changes how much we focus on it. Big issues, big focus, thus no time to look around at the smaller details of life.

When you're caught in the midst of feeling abandoned by God, try to look for His hand in the small things of life again. Now, watch out, because you're bound to encounter more little snags along the way (spilling grape juice on your white shirt, getting stuck in a monstrous traffic jam on the way to a sonogram). Ask God to make you aware of His work in your life during this time. Ask Him to sharpen your spiritual vision. Keep these verses close at hand to remind you of God's promises.

*"So do not fear, for I am with you; do not be dismayed, for I am your God. I will strengthen you and help you; I will uphold you with my righteous right hand"* (Isa. 41:10).

*Jesus said, "And surely I am with you always, to the very end of the age"* (Matt. 28:20).

As Ann and Wallace now realize, "God never left us or laughed at us. He really does love us, and He was showering us with blessings even though we never got pregnant. He wanted us to be totally dependent on Him and to learn how awesome He is. Our faith is the only way we survived infertility and adoption."

**5. Does God still love me? (Because I sure don't feel loved.)**
"The Lord appeared to us in the past, saying: 'I have loved you with an everlasting love; I have drawn you with loving-kindness'" (Jer. 31:3).

After enduring infertility, we couldn't believe that God would then allow our new baby to have significant medical problems. As we left the children's hospital, having learned that Ryan was profoundly deaf, I realized that the previous medical wallops had really taxed my spiritual reserves. This one, though, had sapped the leftovers; I'd never felt more spiritually empty in my life. I broke the stunned silence as we drove home: "You know, Edward, through all the difficulties, I never questioned that God still loved me. But right now, I sure don't feel very loved. God's way of expressing love must be completely different than what I've always thought it was."

I'm still discerning the answer to that realization. I can't tell you precisely how God will tangibly show His love to you, but I do know this: His love is unconditional, unmerited, undeserved, . . . and unending. Jesus Christ is His primary way of showing His love to us. When I start to feel unloved, I make myself remember the unparalleled act of love that God showed to me through His Son. If God never did anything else on my behalf, it was enough that He did that, because He redeemed me for all eternity. But He does more, all the time.

Resolving this question takes some interaction between your head and your heart. Your heart may not feel that God loves you because He's not solving your problem, protecting your pregnancies, or making procedures work. But your head needs to step forward and remind your heart that how God acts in a situation is not the measure of whether or not you are loved by Him. You don't have to *feel loved* to acknowledge that you still *are loved*.

### 6. Is it okay to be angry with God?

Yes, and it's okay to tell Him about it. In fact, it's rather ludicrous not to. God already knows every fragment of thought that crosses your mind—past, present, and future. To not tell Him is just depriving yourself of the freedom to be honest with your Lord. He can handle your outbursts. He's willing to hear your frustrations. He is the safest audience you could ever hope to find.

Anger is a natural reaction to a series of events. If life beats you up long enough, you'll eventually get angry. Your faith wears thin, your emotions rise to the surface, and sometimes what splurts out surprises even you. Where did *that* come from? It came from your deep hurt and disappointment. And God stands ready to listen to every emotion, every comment, every frustration.

"Cast all your anxiety on him because he cares for you" (1 Peter 5:7). Imagine yourself casting it, throwing it, pulling it out from the very depths of your soul, and with great effort, releasing it to God. (For more on dealing with anger, see chapter 6, "Grief: Wandering through the Maze.")

### Communicating with God ... in silence

Like a runner who pulls a hamstring and can only limp along in excruciating pain, infertility cripples your walk with God. Infertility doesn't gallop into your life as a lone rider stirring up trouble. No, it's usually accompanied by problems at work, frustrations with family and friends, tension in your marriage, and personal insecurities. So while you're trying to cure your infertility, you're watching the rest of your life crumble too. *Hello, God? A little attention over this way would be appreciated.*

Infertility may be a hidden problem, but it's not a silent one, at least not for you. It screams at you all day long, bursting back into your thoughts in the middle of anything. Infertility is loud. It drowns out your joy, your peace, your happiness. I truly believe that it's only in the presence of God that you can find peace again. But you have to enter God's presence to find it. You have to take time, make time, to do that.

I look back in my journals to some of the entries from the most intense years of our infertility. I am astonished at what God was teaching me as I stumbled along those rocky paths. My entries were often blunt, raw, and completely honest. Looking back helps me see the big picture of what God was up to.

*I'm tired of being tired. It's not that I don't like my job, because I do. But after eleven-hour days at work, I still don't get caught up. I come home after 7:00 P.M., fall asleep in the recliner, then Edward wakes me up and shuffles me off to bed. And all day, every day, my mind is trying to figure out what to do about having children. I want to find peace—peace with my schedule, peace with my infertility, peace in my walk with God.*

*I keep running across the Luke 10:38–42 passage—in Sunday's sermon, in my editing, in books. God seems to be saying, "Cindy, Cindy, you are worried and upset about many things, but only one thing is needed. Choose what is better, and it will not be taken away from you."*

Jesus told Martha she was too worried about her responsibilities to take time to hear what He was teaching. He'd already elevated women by including them in His teaching sessions, but now He wanted to elevate Martha to another level of life, to give her more than the satisfaction of being a good hostess. He gave her His words of life: "Stop your worries. Sit and listen."

*Today I tried it: Sitting silent before God. I closed my eyes to keep out distractions. But in my mind, I saw myself kneeling, humbling myself before a kind Lord. Wordlessly I lifted up my heart, the center of my emotions and thoughts, for Him to renew and cleanse. So much was packed into it—so many feelings. I gave them all over to Him. Then I offered my entire self . . . and felt His love flood me. Cleansed, made right with Him because His love for me has paid for my sins, I simply desired to receive that which He offered me.*

*My friendship with my Lord is fresh now. The peace I sought rests in my heart. I now feel ready to offer words of love to Him. I offer to God my praise, my love, which sometimes can't be put into adequate words. So I offer my emotions. I "lift up" a feeling to God with a wordless thought, and He knows the depth of that feeling.*

These mostly silent times before God continued for several months. Some days it was easier to quiet the raging noise in my soul than others. I became more comfortable with the silence. It refreshed me to be able to sit in God's presence and just soak up His peace. I became more aware of God's awesome nature. Zephaniah 3:17 says, "He will quiet you with his love."

Remember Philippians 4:7–9? Peace that surpasses our understanding . . . God wants to give that to you. It's not a peace that comes when your infertility is finally cured. It's not a peace that comes from finally attaining parenthood. It's a peace that happens in the midst of the confusion and pain, in the midst of your infertility. It's a relaxing of your soul in the arms of your Lord.

## How other couples have survived spiritually
Linda shares that she and her husband, Olaf, prayed a lot during their seven-year infertility journey, which included two miscarriages plus two failed IVFs. One day Olaf asked her, "When you pray to God about wanting a child, what do you say?" She told him that she asked God to please give them a child. He said he had been praying for peace, asking God to comfort him and to help him overcome these feelings until He was ready for them to have a family. She started praying that way, and "within a few months, I had complete and total peace about my infertility. I was even able to go to baby showers and the mall again."

Paula started looking for things to be thankful for in the midst of her "desert" experience. She found plenty: "I realized we live only twenty minutes from the clinic, while some live three or more hours away. I was thankful my doctor was so knowledgeable, that his staff seemed so personally interested in our case, that we could afford continued treatment, that my prayer partner had experienced and survived infertility, and I even realized I could be thankful that I wasn't barren in biblical times!"

Here are other tips from couples who have been there:
### 1. Be open with God about your feelings, even ugly ones.
He already knows what they are, so not talking to Him honestly only hurts you. But maybe you find it uncomfortable to talk forcefully to God, which is what will probably happen. During some of our deepest valleys, I found it easier to vent to God when there was a lot of noise, such as while vacuuming or while walking on the treadmill. I could talk as loudly as I wanted and not feel inhibited.

### 2. Vent your feelings through journaling.
You may want to keep up with what you're experiencing

medically, but in the long run, you'll be glad you also took time to write what you are feeling right now. Try writing your prayers to God, insights you find in the Bible, and promises He's shown you.

### 3. Strive to stay consistent in your time with God.

Know that every moment you spend with God is like a seed planted that will definitely bear a good harvest in due time. The harvest is that you will be spiritually stronger. But if you never plant seeds, there will be no harvest. Study the stories of couples who have encountered infertility (refer to chapter 13, "Infertile Women of the Bible"). Read the psalms to reassure yourself that your feelings of despair are not a first-time thing. When you find verses of hope and encouragement, put them in prominent places and memorize them.

*Dealing with infertility is certainly a joint effort. All decisions were wrapped in prayer. I was very open to whatever direction God would take us along the way, and I believed strongly that Angela would have a more discerning spirit in this particular crossroad than I would have. I participated in all decisions while being open and receptive to her needs and desires. Little did I realize or know at the time how truly sovereign God is and how His path would not permit us to solve the problem as we saw fit.*      *—Jim*

*God was our rock, our only source of consistency at such an inconsistent time. We spent a lot of time in prayer and Bible study. I know that the strength Keith conveyed was because of God's presence in his life. The only reason I was able to continue to praise God through such a difficult time was because of who He is, not because of who I am. Sure, there were times that we questioned Him—not His complete control, but we questioned His path for us. It's hard to understand the eternal when all we can see is right now. At some very difficult moments, God did give us a peace that literally surpassed all understanding.*      *—Dinah*

Most of all, ask God to use this time of trial to purify you. Ask God to reveal any attitudes or perspectives that need to be changed or adjusted. Be willing to go in the direction He leads.

*Susan and John*

# From abortion to forgiveness

"While we dated, we never really got around to talking about whether or not we would have children when we got married," Susan said. "We never got a chance to answer that question before we found ourselves at an abortion clinic."

Susan's abortion came with multiple levels of complications. She developed an abscess in one fallopian tube, which spread until she had peritonitis. "After having an abortion, I was too scared to go to the campus health center at my Christian college. I almost died before I sought medical help. My fallopian tube had to be removed, and I developed scar tissue from the infection that fused together all my abdominal organs."

She and John eventually married, but then they couldn't conceive. "Obviously we knew we *could* have children, so we suspected that my infertility was a result of the infection and surgery. John didn't want to talk about it. In fact, I had to drag him through the whole infertility process. We wouldn't have any children today if it had been left up to him. He cooperated and was patient only because he knew how much it mattered to me."

For a long time, Susan believed that her infertility was God's punishment for her having had an abortion. "Yet I knew God loved us and forgave us in spite of the fact that we'd had an abortion. I didn't see infertility as vengeance, necessarily, but I knew it was a consequence, a deserved consequence. I don't remember ever doubting God could heal me, but I don't think I ever asked Him directly for mercy or a miracle. I didn't dare. I guess I was hoping that science would find a way around our consequences."

Her remaining fallopian tube was functioning correctly, so they went through the basic tests and the "mildly invasive procedures" to try to find the problem, but nothing showed up. In-vitro fertilization was just being tested, and because of stretched finances Susan and John opted not to try that method. Plus, "we weren't sure what we thought about test tube, petri dish stuff. Was it getting into God's turf? We'd already done that in the past. It just didn't feel right for us."

Eventually, without further medical intervention, and as a total surprise to them and their doctor, they conceived and became parents to Megan. Five years later, Chad was born. "After each child was born, I was hit with a terrible grief as I lay in the hospital, a grief for that other child we'll never know," Susan remembers.

"Infertility is not God's punishment for premarital sex, nor is it a penalty doled out to women who have had abortions. But it can sure feel like it. Although I know I'm forgiven, and I have two children as living proof of God's grace, it's still hard for me to accept forgiveness for those past sins. Infertility may be a consequence of bad choices or bad genes or bad luck, but it is not a punishment from God. There's a big difference between the two. It is important to make that distinction, or else you may find yourself alienated from God when you need Him most."

# Chapter 13

# Infertile Women of the Bible

*As I walked through my infertility journey, I scoured the biblical accounts of barren women for any words of comfort or clues as to how they behaved. I was reassured to see that in case after case, these were righteous, God-fearing women who were not being punished for earlier misdeeds.*

*—Paula*

If infertility is hard to endure in the twenty-first century, think how helpless an infertile woman felt when the nearest fertility clinic was two- to six thousand years down the road. The chief value of a woman in biblical times was first her chastity and, after marriage, her reproductivity.

When I began looking for any woman in God's Word who preceded us in the sisterhood of infertility, names like Rachel, Sarah, and Hannah came to mind quickly, but there were others. What can we learn from each woman? How did she cope with her plight? How did her story end?

Women's names began filling my scribbled pages as I researched the 300-plus women mentioned in Scripture. The most easily identifiable women were barren temporarily, then later blessed with children. In most cases, a woman's barrenness and how God resolved it appeared to be one of the main reasons she was present in Scripture. The point? God used infertility to show His miraculous power and to carry out His plan for human history. These women are described in "Women who were temporarily childless."

The biggest surprise was I could find only one woman who was mentioned as *never* having children—Michal, the first wife of King David. That certainly doesn't mean there weren't more, because surely there were. But the details are missing, so we'll never know who they were. Read Michal's story in this chapter: "A woman who remained childless."

Hannah is the most notable infertile woman in the Bible. We see the depth of her pain physically, emotionally, and spiritually. Hannah's story is told in more detail in this chapter because so many aspects of her plight call to us from the depths of our own pain.

Besides the women discussed in this chapter, many others may have been infertile—their children are never mentioned. Women such as Anna, Jehosheba, Esther, and Miriam may have had children, but Scripture records only who they were and what they did. We should remember that we are more than just bearers of offspring. Women portrayed in the Bible had many important roles, just as we do today.

When I started my research, I intended to title this chapter "*All* the Infertile Women of the Bible," thinking I could compile every woman who struggled with infertility. But digging in, I realized that the lack of details on most biblical women prevented me from discerning whether they were mothers or not. A large number of women are mentioned only once in Scripture. Thus, an absolutely complete list of the infertile women of the Bible will have to remain open-ended. Their stories will remain untold, but the women whose stories we know have spoken to infertile women through the ages.

## Women who were temporarily childless

### Elizabeth
Elizabeth and Zechariah "were upright in the sight of God, observing all the Lord's commandments and regulations blamelessly. But they had no children, because Elizabeth was barren; and they were both well along in years" (Luke 1:6–7). A godly couple, barren, and old—the perfect setting for a miracle! And that's just what happened. While performing his priestly duties, Zechariah was visited by an angel announcing that " 'your prayer has been heard. Your wife Elizabeth will bear you a son, and you are to give him the name John. He will be a joy and delight to you, and many will rejoice because of his birth, for he will be great in the sight of the

Lord'" (vv. 13–15). Elizabeth became the mother of John the Baptist, the long-prophesied one who would prepare the people for the coming of Christ.

Had Elizabeth become a mother in her youth, the news of this postmenopausal baby probably would have been amazing, but not really in the miraculous category. God's plan was to keep her womb closed until both Elizabeth and Zechariah (and everyone who knew them) had given up on their chance of children, and it was precisely the absence of previous children that made the coming of this one so remarkable. After John's birth and naming (complete with a tongue-loosing miracle for the new dad), "the neighbors were all filled with awe, and throughout the hill country of Judea people were talking about all these things. Everyone who heard this wondered about it, asking, 'What then is this child going to be?' For the Lord's hand was with him" (vv. 65–66).

### Manoah's wife, Samson's mother

It's surprising that we're never given this barren woman's name, because her faith is admirable. Twice, an angel appeared to her to provide details of her upcoming pregnancy, and twice the angel explained that she would carry the burden of raising the child in strict accordance to the Nazirite vow, a consecration to God that would begin in the womb for this baby.

Manoah prayed for the angel's second appearance to confirm what his wife had told him, but the angel returned to the woman, not to her husband. She ran and got Manoah, who then asked the angel how they were to raise the boy. "Your wife must do all that I have told her," the angel said, repeating the instructions. She got it the first time, in all likelihood. It appears that Manoah was a little insecure in this divine calling to parenthood (not unlike Zechariah). As the couple was sacrificing a goat, the angel ascended to heaven on flames, leaving Manoah fretting that they would both die after having been so close to seeing God. His wife quickly deduced the situation and calmed him. "If God wanted to kill us, He wouldn't have accepted our burnt offerings nor told us the incredible things that are about to happen."

Pragmatic and faithful, this woman was likely a needed

balance between the high-strung Samson and the pensive, worrisome Manoah. (See Judges 13.)

### Rachel

Young and attractive, Rachel had a lot going for her. She was "lovely in form, and beautiful" (Gen. 29:17). When her never-before-seen cousin Jacob strolled into town (actually, to the field where she watched sheep), it was love at first sight. After only a month, he asked to marry her (29:14, 18). Jacob worked for seven years to earn the right to wed Rachel, only to be tricked into marrying Leah, the "weak-eyed" sister, on the wedding night. Weak-eyed, perhaps, but certainly very fertile. "When the Lord saw that Leah was not loved, he opened her womb, but Rachel was barren" (29:31).

Leah had no marital fulfillment, but plenty of children, while Rachel had her husband's affections but her infertility was driving her crazy. God wasn't doling out barrenness as punishment to Rachel, though we aren't given any clear reasons for her trial. We do see how she responded to them, though. "When Rachel saw that she was not bearing Jacob any children, she became jealous of her sister. So she said to Jacob, 'Give me children, or I'll die!'" (30:1). Basically, she threw a fit. Jacob felt the powerlessness that husbands feel in the battle with infertility. "Am I in the place of God, who has kept you from having children?" (30:2).

Leah eventually birthed six sons and one daughter. Rachel watched them grow up, then watched two servants bear Jacob four sons, a common tradition in that era. With eleven children running around the family tents, "God remembered Rachel; he listened to her and opened her womb. She became pregnant and gave birth to a son, and said, 'God has taken away my disgrace'" (30:22–23). With the birth of Joseph, probably the most doted son in the Bible, her infertility was over. But with the eventual birth of her second son, Benjamin, Rachel knew she was dying as a result of childbirth. In a sad irony, her original, desperate cry came back to haunt her. God granted her the deepest desire of her heart, children, but the very act of producing them robbed her of the opportunity to see them grow to manhood. (See Gen. 29–31; 33; 35; 46; 48.)

## Rebekah

We often forget that Rebekah was at one time infertile. But Genesis tells us in no uncertain terms: "Isaac prayed to the Lord on behalf of his wife, because she was barren. The Lord answered his prayer, and his wife Rebekah became pregnant" (Gen. 25:21). We know nothing of her infertility struggles other than that brief mention. During her pregnancy, she must have been extremely uncomfortable because "the babies jostled each other within her, and she said, 'Why is this happening to me?' So she went to inquire of the Lord. The Lord said to her, 'Two nations are in your womb, and two peoples from within you will be separated; one people will be stronger than the other, and the older will serve the younger' " (vv. 22–23). Her twin sons, Esau and Jacob, defined the term *sibling rivalry* early on, bringing both joy and deep grief to their parents.

Since Rebekah never became pregnant again, we assume her infertility returned, that God closed up her womb again. His broad purposes for Hebrew history required that Rebekah only birth two sons, two nations. (See Gen. 25.)

## Ruth

This incredibly upbeat woman came from a background of heartbreak. Married first to Mahlon, son of Naomi and the late Elimelech, she had no children with him before he died. We don't know how long they were married, but it's safe to say that Ruth married Mahlon in her most youthful years. Bearing children quickly was common, considering there was no birth control other than abstinence (and what newly married couple can manage that?). It's possible Mahlon had infertility issues that kept him from impregnating Ruth. Nevertheless, Ruth knew the heartache of childlessness . . . and widowhood.

After Naomi lost her husband and eventually both sons in the land of Moab, she was left with no means of support and two widowed daughters-in-law. Not a very promising future for any of them. The best answer was to send the young women back to their parents' homes, where they could eventually remarry and have the security and support she couldn't supply.

Ruth refused to leave Naomi and insisted on returning with her to Bethlehem (in the country of Judah), no small journey for two widows traveling alone. The Dead Sea separates Judah and Moab, so the shortest route was to sail across the sea, about 10 miles wide, then walk 15 miles to Bethlehem. To take the land route meant trekking close to 100 miles.

But what would await Ruth when she entered Judah? Hebrew men were strongly discouraged from marrying foreign women. By choosing to remain with Naomi, she was, in effect, risking permanent widowhood and childlessness in order to stay with her beloved mother-in-law. She could have stayed in Moab, married a Moabite, and perhaps had children—a normal life. She showed unparalleled courage and selflessness by choosing a path most young women would refuse.

But perhaps something more caused Ruth to leave her homeland willingly. Moab's idol worship of Chemosh and Molech included horrible rituals of infanticide. Children were made to pass through or into the fire. Excavations have uncovered infant skeletons in burial places around shrines. Maybe she was glad to leave a land in which her offspring, if they had been born, might have been offered on a pagan altar.

The well-known end to this love story is Ruth's marriage to a kind Hebrew named Boaz. Ruth 4:13 says that "the Lord enabled her to conceive," which implies that God acted intentionally, and certainly makes us wonder if Ruth and Mahlon both suffered from infertility problems. Ruth birthed Obed, who fathered Jesse, who fathered King David. So, though childless for a time, Ruth became the great-grandmother of the greatest Jewish king who ever lived. Such a remarkable conclusion deserves one more insight, though. If Ruth had birthed children with Mahlon, she might not have felt compelled to accompany Naomi to Bethlehem with children in tow. Therefore, her temporary childlessness allowed her to freely walk forward into the amazing plan God had waiting for her. (See the book of Ruth.)

*Sarah*
In the midst of a family genealogy and travel history, we first learn of Sarah's predicament: "Now Sarai was barren; she had

no children" (Gen. 11:30). Plain and simple, Sarah was infertile in a time when the world was young, and couples were extremely fruitful. But God took Sarah and Abraham on a long road toward parenthood. Their infertility journey spanned decades, perhaps fifty years or more.

Long bouts of infertility are hard to bear, and we glimpse how downhearted Abraham felt: " 'Sovereign Lord, what can you give me since I remain childless and the one who will inherit my estate is Eliezer of Damascus? . . . You have given me no children; so a servant in my household will be my heir" (Gen. 15:2–3). But all along the way, God was making and repeating His promise to Abraham that he and Sarah would indeed bear a child of their own (Gen. 12:1–3, 7; 13:14–17; 15:4–5, 18–21; 17:1–8). "A son coming from your own body will be your heir," God promised. "Look up at the heavens and count the stars—if indeed you can count them. So shall your offspring be" (15:4–5).

Sarah was a woman whose natural beauty must have been remarkable. Wherever they went, Abraham was afraid other men would kill him to take her (Gen. 12, 20). But Sarah would have traded her looks for fertility any day. So desperate and impatient was she to have a child to call her own, she gave her servant Hagar to Abraham in an ancient kind of biological surrogacy. Sarah could claim any child Hagar bore as her own. Sure enough, Hagar turned up pregnant, but then she began to taunt Sarah.

Sarah's cry sounds just like the emotional irrationality we often feel as we battle infertility. She had instigated Hagar's pregnancy, but then she blamed Abraham for her misery: "You are responsible for the wrong I am suffering. I put my servant in your arms, and now that she knows she is pregnant, she despises me" (16:5). Abraham washed his hands of the matter and told Sarah to deal with her servant however she desired.

In one of the ugliest scenes imaginable, infertile Sarah "mistreated" (physically abused) pregnant Hagar out of anger and deep grief. When we think how agonizing and painful infertility can be, we imagine that poor Hagar took quite a beating that day. She ran to the desert to escape Sarah's wrath. An angel comforted her, telling her she would be the mother of a nation, and sent her back to Sarah with a humble attitude. Hagar birthed Ishmael when Abraham was eighty-six. Sarah never found room in her heart to love Ishmael as her own.

Thirteen years passed. Thirteen more years of infertility, of questioning, of emotional ups and downs. When Abraham was ninety-nine, God had a long conversation with him (Gen. 17), renewing His promise to give Abraham and Sarah a child by the same time next year and establishing with him the covenant of circumcision. During this exchange, "Abraham fell facedown; he laughed and said to himself, 'Will a son be born to a man a hundred years old? Will Sarah bear a child at the age of ninety?' " (17:17). We usually think of Sarah as being the only one who laughed in disbelief, but Abraham did too.

Soon after, Abraham saw three visitors approaching, one of whom was the Lord. The Lord reaffirmed the promise that an heir would be born the next year. Eavesdropping from her tent, Sarah laughed to herself, "After I am worn out and my master is old, will I now have this pleasure?" (18:12). The Lord heard her laughing and gently chided her disbelief.

"Now the Lord was gracious to Sarah as he had said, and the Lord did for Sarah what he had promised. Sarah became pregnant and bore a son to Abraham in his old age, at the very time God had promised him" (Gen. 21:1–2). From God's earlier instructions, they named their newborn "Isaac," which means "he laughs," a clear connection to their laughter upon hearing they would be parents in their old age.

We can imagine that laughter reigned in their home now. The dregs of infertility swept away, Sarah laughed daily as she saw baby Isaac toddling around her tent, tripping over pillows and playthings. And Abraham, though old, found energy to play games like "hide-and-seek" with his son, just for the pleasure of hearing the little boy erupt in squeals of excitement when his daddy found him. Their laughter of disbelief forgotten, they were consumed by the laughter of contentment. (See Gen. 11–23.)

*A personal note: Laughter is the most noticeable thing our Ryan has brought to our home. The pain of our infertility is rarely remembered, now that we have a silly little boy's antics to observe. "Play*

'Where's Ryan?'" he signs, and off we go, running through the
house laughing and surprising each other at every turn. Like
Abraham and Sarah, my husband and I thank God for the laughter
that heals our wounds.

### The Shunammite woman

This unnamed woman and her aging husband had no children, but we get the idea she'd come to a peace about it. One
reason she may have been content without children is
because, with a wealthy husband, she wasn't likely to go hungry in her widowhood. She would be provided for by his
estate, so she didn't worry about whether a child would care
and provide for her as she grew old. Yet she would see God
work three miracles in her life, all related to the child she
thought she'd never have.

The woman showed great kindness to Elisha and his servant as they traveled, providing food and lodging whenever
the traveling twosome came to town. In fact, the woman persuaded her husband to build and furnish an extra room for
Elisha's sole use. She never expected her kindness would reap
lasting rewards.

The first miracle was when Elisha predicted she would
have a child in the next year. She basically said, "Please don't
tease me with this incredible possibility if it's not really going
to happen. I couldn't bear the heartache again." Her words
make us wonder if she'd had plenty of hopes dashed in the
years before and that she'd found peace at last. The mere possibility of a promised baby was enough to send her down the
road of emotional confusion again. (We sure can relate to
that!) As promised, God brought an end to her barrenness—
within a year she was rocking a son in her arms.

The second miracle happened when the boy was out in the
fields with his father. He suddenly began complaining of
headaches. The little boy was brought to his mother, where he
sat in Mama's lap for hours with his head on her chest before
he finally died. Then his mother did something really strange,
but incredibly faithful. She put him on Elisha's bed in the
extra room where no one could disturb his body or even
know he had died. (Not even his father was told, who likely
would have talked her out of her plans.) Then she ran to

Elisha (one commentary estimated Elisha may have been six-teen miles away, three to four hours on foot). She persuaded Elisha to come back with her (another three to four hours), so he went to the boy and restored life to the child.

The third miracle came indirectly. Elisha told the woman that a seven-year famine was coming upon the land, and that she and her family should leave. So they did. When they returned, years later, she was not able to reclaim her house and property. Nothing is mentioned in this passage about her husband. He had probably died. She decided to appeal directly to the king for her rights to the property. Meanwhile, Elisha's servant Gehazi was talking with the king, who was just asking about the great things Elisha had done. Gehazi was recounting the wonders of the prophet's ministry. When he got to the part of the story about how Elisha had restored life to the son of a formerly barren woman, suddenly in walked the woman and her son to plead before the king. "Why, here's the very woman and her son right now!" Gehazi said.

Circumstantial? Maybe. Divinely orchestrated? Definitely. The king was so impressed, he gave her back her land, home, and even paid her for the seven years' income she'd lost by leaving. God's miracle to end her barrenness was one that kept bearing fruit for years afterward. (See 2 Kings 4:8–37; 8:1–6.)

### Tamar

Tamar heads the list of what some people will do to have a baby. She conceived by her father-in-law in order to carry on the lineage of her dead husband. But let's back up: As the wife of Er, Tamar became a young widow because her hus-band was evil, and the Lord ended his life. The custom of the day was that the dead man's brother(s) were next in line to receive the widow so she could conceive by one of them and carry on the lineage of the deceased. But Er's younger brother, Onan, was selfish, and though he fulfilled his duty to sleep with Tamar, he made sure she got none of his semen. God knew of Onan's deceitfulness, so Onan died too. By this time, Judah (son of Jacob, brother of Joseph, father of Er and Onan) probably thought Tamar was bad news. He'd lost two sons in the time she'd been in the family. He had one son left, Shelah, who was too young to marry. So he told Tamar to "live as a widow" (not to remarry) and to wait for Shelah to grow up.

Years passed, and Tamar knew Shelah had come of age, yet Judah hadn't followed through on his end of the deal. So Tamar cooked up a most bizarre plan: When Judah came through town on a sheep-shearing mission, Tamar disguised herself as a prostitute, had sex with her father-in-law, and requested several of his personal items as security until he could send back the payment of a young goat. She didn't care about the goat, but wanted recognizable items that belonged solely to Judah.

Three months later, Tamar's pregnancy was public knowledge. News reached Judah that his widowed daughter-in-law was pregnant, though no one knew by whom. "Burn her," he cried, though why he had a sudden desire to avenge criminal behavior is a mystery. He'd slept with a prostitute and kept it secret. Now he was ready to publicly execute Tamar, which, on one hand, would rid him of the little problem he kept avoiding—his promise to give Tamar to Shelah. With her out of the way, Shelah would be free to marry anyone. He got the surprise of his life when Tamar sent word to him, along with the returned items, that she was pregnant by the man who owned those things. Floored by the revelation of his sin and the lengths to which Tamar went to conceive for Er's sake, Judah called her "more righteous than I" though both of them had some hefty sins to their names. Tamar bore twin boys, Perez and Zerah. Perez's part of the family tree eventually included Christ.

Whether or not Tamar was truly infertile, we don't know. She may have been the victim of bad timing—not being able to have intercourse frequently enough before both Er and Onan died. But for whatever reason, she was determined to get pregnant before her fertile years passed her by. (See Gen. 37–38.)

### Women in the household of the King of Gerar
It's a complicated story, to be sure, but at one time a royal family and staff were stricken with infertility. To start with, Abraham and Sarah lived for a while in Gerar, an area ruled

by King Abimelech. The people weren't known for godliness, and Abraham feared that when men saw how beautiful Sarah was, they wouldn't think twice about killing him and taking Sarah as their own. But if they thought she was his sister, they wouldn't knock him off to get to her.

So Abraham told everyone Sarah was his sister, which wasn't entirely untrue because she was his half sister (same father, different mothers). Though it's hard to imagine, Sarah was about ninety years old and still stunning, which explains why her ageless radiance caught the eye of none other than King Abimelech, who took her into his harem with the intention of sleeping with her. Fortunately, he never got around to it.

At some point, "the Lord had closed up every womb in Abimelech's household because of Abraham's wife Sarah." We don't know how long Sarah was in the king's harem, but it was long enough for people to realize no one was conceiving or bearing children. The truth was revealed when the king had a frightening dream in which God told him Sarah was Abraham's wife and should be returned unharmed.

The king quickly confronted Abraham, who finally 'fessed up to being her husband. Abimelech more than gladly sent them away with one thousand pieces of silver, a handsome sum since a slave cost about thirty. "Abraham prayed to God, and God healed Abimelech, his wife and his slave girls so they could have children again." We're left to wonder if Abimelech was stricken with a physical problem too because we're told "Abimelech had not gone near her." In the dream, God told him, "I have kept you from sinning against me. That is why I did not let you touch her." God may have caused the king to have a physical problem that prevented him from consummating his union with his new acquisition. God used communal infertility to protect Sarah since Abraham was afraid to protect her.

What makes this story even more amazing is that about thirty years earlier, Abraham had pulled the same number on Pharaoh when he tried to make Sarah part of his harem. Fearful for his life, Abraham told the men of Egypt that she was his sister. "But the Lord inflicted serious diseases on Pharaoh and his household because of Abram's wife Sarai" (Gen. 12:17). We aren't told what the diseases were, but the severity caused Pharaoh not to have sex with Sarah (see Gen. 12:10–20). Abraham should have learned to trust God to protect himself and his eye-popping wife the first time.

Ironically, soon after the Gerar debacle, God gave Sarah the pregnancy He had been protecting her for, the son of promise that Abraham had so longed for "at the very time God had promised him" (Gen. 21:2).

## A woman who remained childless

### Michal

Michal was a princess and the wife of a king, but her life was no Cinderella story. The daughter of King Saul, she fell in love with handsome young David, the warrior destined to be king. As a prize for his military success, she was given in marriage to David. Her loyalty was wrapped up in their mutual love, and to protect him she helped him escape Saul's crazed vengeance in one memorable incident (1 Sam. 19).

But once David was in hiding, Saul repossessed her to strike back at David. Unbelievably, Saul gave her to another man, Paltiel. According to one timeline, it was probably about eight years later that David took Michal from Paltiel and claimed her as his wife again. Paltiel was so grieved over losing her that he wept and wailed as he followed behind the entourage.

We don't know if Michal felt the same way about her second husband (2 Sam. 3). The poor woman had been tossed around like merchandise for years, and in the process she developed a sour attitude. Michal is most remembered for her caustic remarks to David when he publicly danced in the streets as the treasured ark of the covenant was brought back to Jerusalem (2 Sam. 6). After David rebuked her, we're left with this somber ending to Michal's presence in Scripture: "And Michal daughter of Saul had no children to the day of her death" (2 Sam. 6:23). As acidic as their words were in their last recorded dialogue, we can safely assume that David and Michal never shared intimacy again. David had other wives (with less emotional baggage) who willingly satisfied his sexual needs.

Nowhere in these passages does it say that Michal was punished by God with infertility. Her barrenness could have been circumstantial. She might not have been married to David long enough the first time to have adequate time to conceive. While she was with Paltiel, she bore no children, but since we have no record of his offspring by other wives, we are left to wonder if he had fertility problems of his own. When reclaimed by David almost a decade later, Michal was older, less fertile, and no longer David's only wife. She watched her sister Merab bear five sons by husband Adriel, plus David's other wives bore him plenty of offspring. Her role as the first wife of David, as well as the daughter of the former king, should have ensured her a degree of exaltation within the king's household. But she was likely looked upon with pity until the day she died. (See 1 Sam. 14:49; 18; 19; 25; 2 Sam. 3; 6; 1 Chron. 15:29.)

## Hannah's story

What a gift God has given us in the story of Hannah! Her eleventh-century-B.C. journey closely resembles the struggles of infertile women in the twenty-first century. She was often consumed by her thoughts of infertility—she went alone to the temple and cried her heart out to God. She made drastic promises to the Lord in hopes she would be given a child. She was stabbed with the pain of watching other women bear children with no problem.

In Hannah, we see a complete picture of the pain of infertility. She was in love with her husband, Elkanah, and longed for children. And adding to her pain was Peninnah, Elkanah's fertile wife, who spoke cruelly to Hannah, taunting her because of her infertility.

Someone probably took Hannah's hand, patted it gently, and advised, "As soon as Elkanah takes a second wife, you'll turn up pregnant. You wait and see. I've seen it happen time and time again." But that hadn't happened. Someone else likely advised, "Stop worrying so much about it. When you stop trying, that's when you'll turn up pregnant." That hadn't happened either. No doubt someone said, "Do you have anything you need to confess before the Lord? Is there a sin you're hiding?"

Maybe Hannah could have lived out her days in security with her husband—if Peninnah hadn't been such a pain to live with. She flaunted her fertility, she berated Hannah's lack of it, and she never ran out of biting comments to toss Hannah's way. Hannah watched in hopeless grief as the fertile Peninnah became pregnant again and again and again.

Hannah tried her best to love Peninnah's children apart from her own grief, and sometimes she could. Who could help but love a tiny infant who asks for nothing more than the warm security of your arms? Looking into the chubby face of the latest family addition, Hannah would watch his eyes close in contented sleep. With very little effort, she could pretend for a few moments that the child was her own, that he was the long-awaited answer to her prayers. But then it would be feeding time, and Peninnah would return to remind Hannah that the baby needed his *mother.*

Every year Elkanah gathered his wives and children for their annual trek to Shiloh for the Feast of Tabernacles, a celebratory time of religious sacrifices, feasting, and observances. The feast was really more of a festival, with people coming from all around the area to commemorate God's care for the Israelites when they were wandering in the desert. Elkanah would share his food with Peninnah and her children, but to Hannah he gave a double portion because he loved her so. He knew how heartbroken she was.

Peninnah was always ugliest during the trips to Shiloh, complaining about the endless responsibilities of mothering all those children on a road trip, griping at Hannah for not helping her more. In Shiloh, Hannah's eyes flooded every year when she found herself surrounded by so many women with children in tow—exhausted mothers who snapped at their children, young mothers with twins nursing at each breast, older mothers who never seemed to stop bearing children. The annual festival was the only time she saw many of these women from other villages, and every year too many of these women had birthed another child since she had last seen them.

One year Hannah reached the end of her emotional rope. Peninnah had poked and prodded her ruthlessly, even while they were at the Lord's house. Hannah cried so much that she couldn't eat. Elkanah tried to comfort her, begging her to eat and to perk up. He meant well when he said, "Don't I mean more to you than ten sons?" To have seven sons was the greatest blessing for a Jewish woman—seven symbolized completeness—but to birth ten sons would have made her nothing less than an icon among her peers. Of course, Elkanah was the love of her life, but another part of Hannah ached for a child with such a longing that it threatened to rip her soul in two.

Depressed and feeling completely alone in her grief, Hannah sought out the Lord's house, where the agony of her soul split the silence of the room. In this private moment with her Lord, Hannah's cries erupted from every part of her being. She was determined to vent it all this very day, to pour forth the anguish until her soul could rest in quiet exhaustion. She found herself praying as she'd never prayed before, pleading and making vows to her God that she swore she would keep at all costs. As she prayed her lips moved, but her voice was silent. She had no need to voice the words she knew her Lord could hear. It was a startling moment of intimacy between Hannah and her God, born from years of heartache.

Infertile women have been making bargaining-type promises to God for generations. Hannah knew you don't make promises to God that you don't plan to keep. Yet, in this moment before the Lord she felt it right to beg God for a son who would be useful to His service.

"Oh, God," she pleaded, "look upon your servant's misery and remember me in the months to come. Don't forget about my pleas for a son. I'll give him back to You as Your servant for his entire life. I won't count him as my son first, but will always look at him as Your servant first, and my son second."

Eli, the priest, watched this lone woman carefully. He'd heard her wails and tears mixed with interludes of silence. He'd seen others come in and out of the temple in all sorts of conditions—some drunk, some with guilt written all over them. Not everyone who came to town for the feast lived righteous lives the other weeks of the year. He wondered what this woman's story was. Her cries sounded unintelligible, as if she'd hit the wine flask a little too heavily. Time for a little priestly intervention.

Hannah was startled when she heard Eli's footsteps approaching, so immersed was she in her prayerful pleading.

"Woman, enough of this getting drunk and stumbling into the temple," he said, on the verge of impatience. "How long will you let your drinking go uncontrolled?"

*What in the world is he talking about?* Hannah wondered. Then it hit her. Her cries must have sounded like the wails of the drunk women she'd seen staggering down Shiloh's streets. With a quick swipe across her wet cheeks, Hannah proved herself by her clarity of thought and speech.

"Not so, my lord," she said. "Don't mistake me for a wicked, drunken woman. I've not poured myself anything to drink, but instead I've poured out my soul to the Lord. I've been here praying from the depths of my anguish and grief."

So private had her conversation been with God that she hesitated to tell Eli the requests and pledges she'd vowed before her Lord. Fortunately, the priest didn't inquire further, but instead offered her a blessing and reassurance.

"Go in peace, then" he said, with a new look of gentleness on his face. "And may the God of Israel give you what you have asked for."

Did he mean it? Her heart soared! After hours of pouring out her anguish to her Lord, pleading and searching her soul, she now let the priest's words flow into her heart, bringing with them a sense of comfort she hadn't felt in years. She felt so clean inside—even the wounds from Peninnah's assaults didn't hurt anymore. And what was this other thing she felt? Could it actually be *hope*?

Elkanah knew something was different when Hannah returned. For one thing, her face was the prettiest he'd seen it in a long time, even if her eyes did look a little puffy. But the smile on her face was genuine, and she even mentioned wanting to find something to eat. Maybe the Hannah he used to know was coming back after all!

The next morning the entire family gathered their belongings for the return trip to Ramathaim. Peninnah was in a foul mood as usual, made even more so by the fact that her sharp tongue didn't even make Hannah flinch. No one could dislodge the peace Hannah felt.

Months passed. Hannah tried to be patient for what she believed God would bring about. Then one day she was sure. She was absolutely sure she was pregnant. Her happiness knew no bounds! When she told Elkanah, he reacted with all the joy she ever imagined he would. But she had something more to tell him. She had to tell him about her pledge, her vow before God when they were back in Shiloh.

She revealed to her husband her promise to God: If He would remember her by giving her a son, she would give that son back to the Lord to be a servant for his entire life. She would consecrate this child with the Nazirite vow—a pledge that separates a person for God's use (Num. 6:1–21).

Elkanah was probably speechless. The Nazirite vow was strict. Some people consecrated themselves with a Nazirite vow for short periods of time, but his wife had consecrated their unborn child for life. She would never cut his hair, never let him taste a fermented drink, never even let him eat the grapes or raisins used to make wine. She would keep her child away from the corpses of dead people until he was old enough to do it himself. Elkanah knew that the Nazirite vow was not generally the kind of vow that someone, like a mother, took for their child; it was a vow a person voluntarily took upon him- or herself.

He also knew that as a Jewish man he had the legal right before God to revoke his wife's pledge. God had given Moses the instructions that were passed down from generation to generation, and every Jew knew that a woman's pledge could be overridden by her father or her husband (Num. 30). With one word, Elkanah could forbid her pledge on behalf of their son, and God would release Hannah entirely. On the other hand, if Elkanah said nothing upon learning of the vow, then the vow would stand. God would hold her—*and Elkanah*—responsible for keeping the vow. Elkanah would become a participant if he said nothing to revoke it.

Whether Elkanah pondered his response quickly or slowly, we don't know. But he decided to stand in agreement with his beloved Hannah, committing himself to uphold the vow with her. That he respected her pledge before God says volumes about his love for his wife, about his trust in her relationship with God, and about the strength of his own faith. It meant

Elkanah wouldn't see his son daily once he was old enough to serve in the temple. It meant doing something that no one else would understand or agree with. But Elkanah let his wife's pledge stand. And he stood beside it.

When her child was born, Hannah named him Samuel because "I asked the Lord for him." The name Samuel sounds like the Hebrew phrase "asked or heard of God." (*El* is Hebrew for "God.") News spread from house to house and from village to town that the once-barren Hannah had birthed a son—*and* that she had made a radical promise to God—*and* that Elkanah had not revoked her pledge. How tongues must have wagged!

Hannah spent the next several years nursing her baby. In that culture, children were often nursed for three or more years. Samuel went from infant to toddler to little boy. When Elkanah and Peninnah and their brood made the journey to Shiloh each year, Hannah didn't go in those early years of Samuel's life. In her heart, she knew the next time she went to Shiloh, it would be to present Samuel before the Lord and leave him under Eli's tutelage.

The years passed, and all too quickly little Samuel was old enough to live at the temple. What an incredible moment it must have been in the lives of Hannah and Eli when she told the old priest, "I am the woman you thought was drunk that day. I prayed for this child, and God has answered. So now I give my son to the Lord for his whole life." Surely Eli, a man whose own sons were known for ungodliness, must have marveled at the faith of a woman who would keep a promise like that.

We can wonder how she, who had waited so long for a child, could bring herself to turn over her energetic, inquisitive little boy to the care of an aging priest. But we find our answer in her prayer of praise before the Lord (1 Sam. 2:1–10). "My heart rejoices in the Lord; in the Lord my horn is lifted high. . . . There is no Rock like our God." Having your horn lifted up by God symbolizes being delivered from disgrace to honor and strength. Her poetic praise has been called the Magnificat of the Old Testament, paralleling the song of praise that Mary, the mother of Jesus, gave in the New Testament (Luke 1:46–55). Hannah went on to testify that God was in the business of turning emptiness into fullness, sadness into joy, longing into satisfaction. "Those who stumbled are armed with strength. . . . Those who were hungry hunger no more. She who was barren has borne seven children. . . . He raises the poor from the dust and lifts the needy from the ash heap; he seats them with princes and has them inherit a throne of honor."

*Hannah found her source of joy in her Lord, not in her child.* God answered her prayer and she answered her pledge.

Undoubtedly, it was hard for Hannah to leave her boy at the temple when it was time for the family to return to their village. Little Samuel's bottom lip probably quivered. Maybe he cried and ran to hug her again. Hannah's heart was on the verge of breaking. But she called upon the faith that had caused her to make that pledge in the first place—if God was big enough to give her a child, then He was big enough to watch after her little boy at the temple. And He was big enough to comfort a mother's heart.

We catch glimpses of Hannah in other annual trips to Shiloh. Surely no one looked forward to those trips more than Hannah! But never did she ask Samuel to come home. Each year she took her growing son a new robe she'd sewn by hand. Imagine how she must have prayed for her son with each and every stitch. Those robes were laced with the prayers and love of a mother whose faithfulness to God has testified through the centuries.

Eli surely had a special word of blessing for Elkanah and Hannah each year. They certainly distinguished themselves from the crowds who came and went in the annual processions. Eli asked God to give them more children since they had given their son to the Lord. And God did just that. Hannah gave birth to three sons and two daughters. Her life had once been marked by barrenness. Now her world was full of her own children, and she could walk through every day knowing she'd kept a remarkable promise to God.

Samuel's long life as a priest before God was remarkable too. He was purely devoted to his God, as few others have ever been. His prophetic insights from the Lord guided Israel for decades. God used Samuel to anoint the first and second kings of Israel, Saul and David. Samuel's life of consecration had been set in motion before he was even conceived—because his mother, Hannah, was a barren woman of great faith.

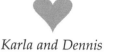

*Karla and Dennis*

# *Miracles in spite of infertility*

Even after trying whatever is medically available to overcome infertility, there are still couples who find that nothing helps them conceive. But sometimes, when the specialists can do no more, God works a miracle. Karla and Dennis know from experience.

After a year of trying to conceive with no success, Karla went to her ob/gyn. He started her on temperature charts, checked her fallopian tube (one had been removed due to an earlier infection), and ordered a round of tests and procedures for both Karla and Dennis.

"Nobody could say why we were having trouble. Everything seemed to be working. We took some time off to look at our options, including adoption."

It was the spring of 1983, and Karla decided to resign her marketing/public relations job in order to pursue some freelance work. Then in July Dennis lost his job when his division closed. "We went from two incomes to no income! And no insurance. We didn't even address the infertility subject all summer. We were in survival mode."

At the end of the summer, Karla was sick with what she thought was the flu. "Our next-door neighbor was a cute little guy who was like a brother to us. He was in our kitchen one morning and I was lying on the window seat, telling him how wretched I felt. He said, 'I think you're pregnant. My sister's pregnant, and she has all the same symptoms.' I told him how ridiculous that was."

But later that week, the Thursday before Labor Day, Karla went to the fertility clinic for a pregnancy test. "Those home pregnancy tests were still very new and nobody trusted them yet!" Because of the holiday weekend, Karla was told not to expect a call until the following Tuesday. "But on Friday, just before their office closed, the nurse called me and said, 'I couldn't make you wait all weekend! You'll have to go back to your ob/gyn because we're kicking you out of our program!'"

Karla's doctor was equally amazed that she had become pregnant without medical intervention. "He said, 'Well, it beats me!' We all laughed . . . and we thanked God."

Dennis and Karla's first son, Seth, was born in April 1984. "He was truly a gift, a gift from God." Not daring to expect another miracle, Karla and Dennis were just as surprised to birth Matt six years later. Then Ben was born two years after that.

When Ben was two, Karla had to have a hysterectomy. Her doctor said, "I can't believe we're removing these parts when we had so much trouble getting them to work!" During the surgery he found so much scar tissue and organ damage that he later told her it truly was a miracle that any of her organs worked at all.

Remember the passage in Luke, when Mary and Joseph encountered some very excited shepherds visiting the newborn Jesus? "Mary treasured up all these things and pondered them in her heart" (Luke 2:19). Karla has some unforgettable memories of her own.

"I'll never forget how, at every one of our children's births, my doctor held them up and thanked God for them because they were quite literally miracles. And he prayed for the day they would be born-again. That prayer has been answered for all three."

# Chapter 14

# *When Someone You Know Is Infertile*

*There is absolutely no way to console a couple experiencing infertility. It is so hard to endure. However, when someone says they're praying for you, they're doing the most awesome thing they can do for you.*
 — Linda and Olaf

Bumping along on a minibus, we made the ten-minute jaunt from the airport to our parking lot. It was about 11:00 P.M., we just wanted to drive home and fall into bed. Ryan was way past his bedtime, but he was still going strong.

All six passengers on the minibus sat facing each other, but no one bothered talking. I noticed the couple across from us. The wife's hands clung to her husband's arm. Their silence surprised me a little because people almost always make small talk about Ryan's sign language, and he was busily signing to Edward about this bus adventure—the driver, the chairs, the windows, the lights. Maybe the couple was just as tired as we were, I thought, or maybe they just weren't interested in children.

The driver pulled up to their parking spot first, and the couple unloaded their luggage. As the bus pulled away, Edward looked at me and said quietly, "They're infertile."

"What?!" I certainly never expected this observation from a boring little bus ride. "How do you know?"

"Even though it's dark, I could see she had tears running down her face," Edward said. "She kept watching Ryan. I didn't know what to say. I didn't know whether I should bring it up."

We arrived at our car, loaded our luggage, and hoped the other couple might drive in our direction as they left the parking lot. We wanted to tell them we knew how they felt. We wanted them to know that we'd survived infertility. We wanted to listen to their hurt, if they chose to share it. We wanted them to know they are not alone.

But we never saw them again. They were gone, and with them they carried the image of our happy family of three. They never knew that we understood their pain or that the creation of our family had come after many years of waiting. They will never know how much we wanted to share their grief.

### What to do? What to say?
Maybe it's not a quick encounter on a bus that concerns you. You're wondering what to say to your longtime friend who's been trying to have a child for months, maybe years. Or maybe you've just learned by chance of a couple's struggles, since they appear to everyone as just a childless couple who don't ever talk about having children of their own.

Have you wondered what is the right thing to do or say? This chapter provides you with tips on what to do and what not to do. Don't expect the person battling infertility (male or female) to know how to tell you what they need you to do or say. The upheaval of the experience is so overwhelming that most people don't have the presence of mind to know how to ask for what they need—they're struggling to survive day to day. These ideas were gleaned from couples who have survived infertility and, in retrospect, can see what has made a difference in their lives and relationships when people have tried (successfully or not) to minister to them.

But don't read this chapter only. That's like eating the cherry off a sundae and ignoring the ice cream, syrup, and sprinkles. Read the other chapters to gain deeper insights about infertility from those who know personally.

### Offer empathy, not sympathy
To minister meaningfully, we need to find ways to connect with someone else's pain. This isn't some corny admonition to conjure up falsely empathetic feelings. The truth is, you can never know the pain a particular infertile couple is feeling. Even if you had your own infertility experiences, you can't precisely know theirs. Every situation is different and every

person's way of handling difficult emotions will vary too. But you can draw from your experiences to create a frame of reference for your ministry.

You've heard the terms *empathy* and *sympathy*, but do you know the difference? *Empathy* means to understand another person's feelings by finding something in your life that parallels their emotions. *Sympathy* means to feel sorrow for another's pain without really identifying with it.

Edward is an ordained minister with accredited clinical pastoral education training. He was a hospital chaplain for several years. During that time he was taught to quickly assess how to empathize (not sympathize) with the patient in a hospital room: "Whether that patient is facing chemotherapy, heart surgery, or just outpatient surgery, chaplains have to find a place in their emotional tapestry to help them relate to the patient. They have to find a way to dig down into their own experiences and discover what was most painful. That brings about the ability to empathize. For example, I may not have lost a sister, but I remember the loss of my grandmother.

"Empathy says, 'I've felt what you're feeling in a similar moment, and I know how that experience felt, so to the best of my ability I can minister to you from that perspective.' Sympathy says, 'I'm sorry for you. I have no idea what you're feeling, but I feel sorry for you because of what you're feeling.' There's an air of aloofness about sympathy, and that doesn't bring about ministry. Ministry means coming alongside and saying, 'Let me go *with* you through this,' not 'Let me stand on the outside and pat you on the hand while you're going through this.'"

To try to understand what infertility feels like, take a trip through your own memories. Have you lost a child? You can draw from the pain of that grief experience to empathize with someone experiencing infertility. If you have children, try remembering what it was like when you learned you were expecting a baby. Remember telling your spouse, your parents, your sister, your best friend. Remember the affirmation and encouragement you received from everyone who rejoiced with you over the coming baby.

Remember how pregnancy changed your body, just a little at first, and then so much that you wondered if you'd ever be able to keep any of your former clothes. Would your ankles go back to normal? Remember how you reacted when you first felt the baby kick. Remember the joy of having that newborn placed in your arms for the first time.

Now strip yourself of all those climactic moments. Imagine being deprived of the splendor of having that child placed in your arms. Imagine someone coming up and taking the child away from you. Place your hand on your abdomen and try to imagine what it must feel like to know there will never be a new life growing in there. Think about the loss of knowing you could never feel the kick of a tiny baby's foot or its movement in response to your voice.

Let the hurt reach way down deep. If it brings you to tears, then you're making progress. If it feels like your heart is being ripped from your body, then you're gaining some understanding of what infertility feels like.

Imagine standing at a tiny grave. Your child. Your tiny baby. You'll never know what it feels like to have that child's arms around your neck. You'll never be able to rock him to sleep, feel his warmth against your heart, smell his fresh baby breath, or kiss his little forehead. You'll never know what that baby would look like as a first-grader or at the senior prom. You'll never hear your child's voice or look in her eyes. For that matter, your beloved infant never got to look into your eyes to see your love for him.

Infertility feels like a grave that follows you around. The grave keeps grabbing more and more of your dreams. Infertility is the death of a child you never knew, a child you could never conceive or the baby that your body miscarried. Infertility brings grief in the same way that death brings grief to the survivors. But our society doesn't acknowledge infertility in the same manner as we acknowledge death. People think, *How can you lose what you've never had?*

An infertile couple feels grief as if it were prolonged death. Their hopes soar, then plummet with each failed fertility treatment, with each month that doesn't bring pregnancy. For a few days or weeks they embrace hope, anticipating that surely *this time* they'll be on the road to parenthood. Their minds race forward to all the dreams that seemed out of their reach. Surely *this time* it will all be theirs. But then it all comes crashing down and the dreams die all over again.

To truly care for your infertile friend, you have to explore the recesses of your soul that have likely never been touched. But your emotional awareness will equip you to listen to another person's pain in ways you've never done before. Listen as if it were *your* pain.

## Never assume anything

Several years into our infertility struggles, an acquaintance overheard me talking about adoption possibilities. "*You* want children?" she said with no small amount of surprise. "I always thought you two just weren't interested since you both have careers."

My heart flinched at the familiar stab, the wound that never healed. We didn't make public prayer requests out of our forays into infertility treatments; so of course, not everyone knew we were hoping for a child. Our families and closest friends knew, but this person didn't.

Assumptions are so dangerous. They inflict slow-healing wounds. Never assume the childless couples in your circle of friends are not interested in becoming parents. Never assume their lack of discussion on the topic of childbearing means they have no personal interest. Some couples can't bring themselves to openly share their intimate struggles with anyone, not even close friends.

If you want to gently find out where someone is along the Richter scale of family planning, there are better ways to learn than by asking, "So when are *you* going to have kids?" or "Do you guys want kids or not?" Those questions can set off emotional earthquakes.

A kinder, gentler inquiry is "Are you hoping children will be part of your future?" This allows the person to respond by calling on his or her sense of hope. The word *want* is difficult for the infertile person to hear. His sense of wanting children is so deeply rooted that when someone questions if he *wants* children, it's like a slap in the face, an insult to his personhood. Calling upon his sense of hope lifts their spirit and allows him to share that hope with you: "Oh yes, we hope to have children in our home! We've been praying for a child for two years now."

**Zip your lips (and use your ears)**
To be a true friend to an infertile person, you'll stand out in the crowd if you'll let her cry on your shoulder, talk out her pain, or simply vent her frustration. The old adage holds true: God gave us one mouth and two ears so we would listen twice as much as we talk.

Everyone has advice for an infertile couple. Everyone, from parents to nosy neighbors, thinks he or she can offer something she's read, heard, or something *she thinks* she's read or heard—some big piece of helpful news. Infertility information is everywhere—from the Internet to televised news reports to zany portrayals in movies to magazine features about high-tech babies. No couple involved with fertility treatments is at a loss for information.

I heard the same advice countless times: "Try boxer shorts." "Drink more water." Some people genuinely try to offer suggestions (though it usually isn't based on anything medically sound), while others are just spouting off some remnant of advice they picked up somewhere, as if it's their duty to tell me *something* that might help.

It hurts every time an infertile couple receives advice from someone who really hasn't been in their shoes, when someone gallops in with an answer to their infertility. It makes them feel angry, sad, and frustrated, all at the same time. You'll never know how many private tears are cried over all the advice they endure. In a way, all those helpful hints make a woman and her husband feel like failures all over again, as if the advice giver is saying, "You're not really smart enough to figure this out on your own, so let me help you out." This sounds harsh, but unless you've been in their shoes and have had to receive such advice, you have no idea how horrible the advice makes you feel.

**Listen with a high IQ "involvement quotient"**
Edward has learned much from his experiences as a hospital chaplain. "Many people ask me how I can minister daily to families in the worst of situations. I've seen a preschooler who died from a gunshot wound inflicted accidentally by a cousin. I've watched a little boy die as he waited to receive a heart transplant. The secret is to listen—listen with your heart, your

mind, your soul to what the grieving person is saying to you."

You innately use various levels of listening in your life. At times, you listen intensely to a speaker when the subject hits you square between the eyes. Other times, you listen to the radio, drive, and plan a grocery list in your head. You listen to a friend rattle on about something trivial and only catch part of it.

If you have a friend who is infertile, a friend who trusts you enough to share any part of her or his painful journey, then do your friend a favor and listen intently, as if it were your own problem. Listen as if you were required to accurately summarize the content back to the speaker. Listen well: there are precious few who actually bother listening at all.

Don't assume that your friend has *anyone else* to discuss it with openly because there's a strong chance she doesn't. Most of the women who have shared their stories with me admit that they felt completely alone in their infertility struggle. Most men don't discuss it with their friends, so they feel isolated too.

We can't assume that the couple can vent sufficiently to each other because this isn't always so. An infertile couple is in the epicenter of storm, and each spouse needs someone outside the storm to talk to. They're trying to survive; they know the problem intimately. They talk to each other, but they can't listen in the way that an outside friend can.

Remember, your friend may repeat herself from time to time. It may sound like she keeps beating herself up over the same hurts or frustrations. She may take two steps forward and three steps back. She may seem emotionally confused. She probably cries a lot. A man or woman facing infertility needs you to convey that you're praying, even though the answers aren't coming quickly. Each needs to be reassured that you've heard what he or she has said, that you've listened to and care about the important details.

**Take the initiative to stick by your friend over the long haul**
Too many people ask an infertile couple how they're doing, what treatments they're pursuing, and how they can pray for them. And that's it. There's little or no follow-up.

*I didn't share my experiences with many people, so most had no idea we were even trying to have children. The last two miscarriages we kept to ourselves because the heartache was just too much. I didn't want people feeling sorry for me, especially after losing my best friend. She sensed my pain and couldn't deal with it, so she stopped calling me. I felt as if she had betrayed me. It was then that I realized that some people are uncomfortable being around childless couples.*
                 —Debbie

As someone who cares for an infertile friend, *initiate* discussion regularly. You can't simply say, "Call me if you need to talk," and expect that no news is good news. You can't assume that things are improving simply because she doesn't bring it up during the Sunday School prayer request time. Call your friend at least weekly. Call more often if you can. Risk being a nuisance because you care that much.

It's too easy for an infertile person to feel rejected by friends who don't seem to want to invest time in them. Infertility plays with emotions in strange ways—we imagine that people are ignoring us when perhaps they aren't. We feel that we're excluded from events or conversations because we think people see we're not as much fun to be with. Maybe people don't want to be with us because they think we're an emotional basket case now. Maybe they think we don't want to go to lunch with them because they have kids and we don't. A woman's powers of reasoning may go out the window when she's infertile.

Your friends need you to be with them through the ups and downs, the hills and valleys. Expect a lot of valleys. Stick with them anyway.

### Ask questions gently and only if permitted

When you discover your friend or family member is encountering infertility problems, begin by asking if he or she would like to talk about it, indicating that you're willing to listen and share their pain. They may need you to prove you're willing to listen. Most people just want to listen once or twice, and then they don't ask again. Asking your friend some questions may help him or her feel comfortable, that you're in this for the long haul—that you're a friend who won't go away.

Give her a chance to tell you what she knows. Here are some suggestions for initiating conversation.

- *If you don't mind talking about it a little more, I'm willing to listen.*
- *How long have you realized you've been struggling with infertility?*
- *How are you doing emotionally in all this?*
- *How is your husband doing? How is your wife handling this?*
- *Have you seen a fertility specialist yet? What does he/she recommend?*
- *Have you shared this with either your parents or your spouse's parents?*
- *Are you feeling undue pressure from anyone to become parents?*

Your gentle words of kindness and concern will not go unnoticed or unappreciated.

### Think about how they feel in group settings

Infertile couples agree: One of the hardest things to endure is sitting in a large group that openly discusses the adventures of their own children.

Groups of adults do this all the time—in Sunday school, in missions groups, in clubs, in fellowships, and more. Talking about kids is a natural part of life, and we who are infertile understand that. It's not that we want you to abruptly stop talking about your families in front of us. But a little balance would be nice.

My husband reminded me of our Sunday School class from several years ago. About seven couples were there every week, and three of those couples were trying to conceive. Almost every Sunday, though, the teachers (who had battled infertility themselves) included funny illustrations about their preschoolers. Sometimes the teacher posed a question for discussion, requiring input from people who had no common frame of reference: "Think of a time when your children refused to obey you." We were shocked and hurt that the teachers disregarded the emotions of half the class. How could they have so quickly forgotten the pain of their own infertility? We realize now that we should have gently addressed the teachers, pointing out that their illustrations were alienating the infertile couples. But we didn't. We just sat there, frustrated.

Another pain in the conversational neck is when group conversations turn toward jokingly complaining about children or the tasks of parenthood:

*"My two-year-old has been driving me crazy lately."*
*"Now that my kids are teenagers, I think I'll just put them in a closet until they turn eighteen."*
*"When I think of all the time I used to have before we had kids! What I wouldn't give for a little of that time now."*

When words like these are tossed around, many infertile couples find the only way to survive the pain is to sit in stone-cold silence until the conversation is over. They may want to run from the room, but propriety keeps them in their seats. She tries to stifle the sobs clenching her throat. His mind races between his own sorrow and trying to think of a way to protect his wife from the agony of listening to such comments.

What can you do if a conversation has turned into a swap meet for cute kid stories (or a gripe session)? You can be an ally simply by making eye contact with the couple and trying to convey through your expression that you know it's hurtful to them. Then, jump into the conversation and turn its focus toward something that will be easier for everyone in the group.

### Reach out tangibly to your friend
A couple battles infertility every day, 24/7. Thoughts of inadequacy and frustration are never far removed from their consciousness. It is at times exhausting.

Here are some concrete ways to help them:
• *A warm, sincere hug is better than most anything you can say.* After one of those horrible experiences in a group discussion, be sure to hug your friend. When you've just finished lunch and he's poured out his latest frustration and anger over failed fertility procedures, give him a hug and remind him that you'll continue to pray. When you see her in the church

hall on Mother's Day (or any day), give her a hug and tell her you care about her.

• *Pray for them, pray with them.* It doesn't have to be a twenty-five-minute prayer, but just the act of going the extra mile means so much. If you're together for lunch, include a sentence or two during the meal's blessing. If you've got him on the phone or out for a game of hoops, initiate a brief prayer by saying, "I know you and Kim are really going through a lot. Do you mind if I pray for you real quickly?" If you ride to a retreat together, an extended, conversational prayer time can be a healing and upbuilding experience.

*Don't try to encourage us out of our grief. Don't say, "This is God's will. God wants to teach you something." One woman told us, "I know what it's like to lose children; I've lost animals." Just put your arms around us and tell us you're praying. Cook us a meal once in a while. Send us a note telling us we're not alone. Meet the physical needs of those who are grieving: mow their lawn, clean their house, wash their dishes. Julie received flowers from a family in the church. Those were the things that meant the world to us.*

*—Joe and Julie*

• *When a couple miscarries, remember the date when the baby was due.* One of the hardest parts of miscarriage is coming upon the day the baby was due. No one remembers it except the couple, and they don't feel the freedom to make a big deal of it with others. So they grieve alone. Several times I've made a note in my calendar when a couple's baby was due. When a miscarriage has occurred, I will then send them a note the week of the due date to let them know their baby is not forgotten. You might say

*"I know this week is hard since your precious child was due to make his or her appearance in the world. I just want you to know that your little one has not been forgotten. How I would have loved to meet your baby! How I wish I could watch you hold that baby in your arms! Your child's place in our family will always be missed. You are dear friends to me, and I am praying especially for you as you pass through this valley."*

Make it a note with one purpose only: to comfort them in their grief. Don't trivialize the significance of their child's due date by including general updates about how your job is going, how your kids are doing, or where you just went on vacation. Let your message of loving concern stand alone. Also don't try to explain away their grief with comments like "But we can rest in the assurance that God knows best." Allow them to grieve, and love them through it.

**What to say and what not to say**
The Bible isn't kidding when it says that the tongue can't be tamed. "It is a restless evil, full of deadly poison. With the tongue we praise our Lord and Father, and with it we curse men, who have been made in God's likeness" (James 3:8–9).

I'm not sure I've ever met anyone who innately knows the right things to say unless they themselves have experienced infertility. It can take days to get over the pain inflicted by some people's well-meaning, spur-of-the-moment comments. The memories of some of these thoughtless remarks never go away.

What are some helpful things to say? Surprisingly, the couples I interviewed had very few specific suggestions. What means the most, in their opinion, is the manner in which someone relates to an infertile couple.

*There aren't any good things to say to an infertile couple other than "I love you and I'm praying for you." Really, I felt the less they had to say, the better.* —Ann

*The most helpful thing was a friend who just let me pour out my heart, over and over and over again. She cried with me when I cried, laughed with me (and at me) when I went into my sarcastic mode, helped me to laugh at myself, prayed for me and with me, and was basically just willing to listen. She walked my road with me. At the time she had no understanding of what we were going through, but she was willing to share my burden. It was no surprise to God, but I later walked the road of infertility with her, and we already had a great foundation to build on.* —Angela

However, couples had plenty to offer for a list of things *not* to say. For the sake of those who are battling infertility or who have battled it, read this section carefully, then share it with others!

### Please don't tell an infertile couple

*"You just need to relax."*
Relaxation has nothing to do with conception. The flippancy of this comment implies that a couple's infertility problems really have no medical basis, that it's all in their heads, that they're just too uptight. This comment insults them because it undermines the problem and their emotional struggles.

*"Has your husband tried boxer shorts?"*
Yes, we've all heard this one, and we don't need to hear it again. Just trust the couple to discuss this option with their doctor if they have questions about it. Honestly, do you really want to discuss men's underwear?

*"Take my children for a while— that'll change your mind about having kids!"*
First of all, they don't want *your* children; they want their own! People say this all the time. Though it's always meant as a joke, it's frequently tossed out in the presence of the children, which can't do anything good for their self-esteem. This sad attempt at humor is never very funny.

*"Having kids isn't all it's cracked up to be."*
Maybe not for you, but the infertile couple wants (and deserves) to find this out for themselves. This comment implies that once they have kids, they'll regret it, or they'll look back on their childless years with longing. Don't count on it. We value what we work hard to obtain, and this couple is working very hard to bring a child into their lives.

*"You already have one child. You should be content."*
Couples with secondary infertility (they have one child, but are unable to bear a second) are caught between two worlds.

They don't fit completely with the infertile ranks because childless couples look at them as outsiders, and they don't fit in with those who bear children easily. It's a difficult position to be in, and they receive little or no comfort from anyone, anywhere. Celeste, who had one successful pregnancy in between her miscarriages, said the second miscarriage was much worse than the first. The second time, she knew how incredible it was to have a baby, so she was very aware of all the joy she was missing.

*"Isn't it funny how people who want children can't have them and people who don't want more have a bunch?"*
We can only hope this isn't really an example of the speaker's sense of humor. This situation isn't funny at all, but another reminder of how unfair and unjust life can be, which is a big issue that infertile couples struggle with. The Bible tells us that God "causes his sun to rise on the evil and the good, and sends rain on the righteous and the unrighteous" (Matt. 5:45).

*"When you stop trying, you'll get pregnant."*
Don't we wish?! The statistics have shown again and again that the average couple who has unprotected intercourse with no intentional timing will, over the course of a year, get pregnant. After a year, it's time to see a doctor. Those who actually pay attention to the calendar (i.e., those who *try* to get pregnant) aren't jinxing themselves into infertility. In fact, once the doctors start investigating the problem, one of the first things a couple will do is have intercourse very frequently and very intentionally during periods of ovulation. In other words, the doctors will have them try harder for a little while.

*"Just remember, God works all things together for good."*
This has to be one of the most overused, misunderstood comments in Christendom, and it's tossed around for everything from untimely death to flat tires. And it usually is spoken while the person pats your hand or shoulder. It's true that "God works for the good of those who love him" (Rom. 8:28), but that verse does not say that all things *are* good. The comment pushes the hearer to hurry up and call infertility *good*. "Now I'm supposed to think all this pain is *good* for me?"

That's much too painful a leap for a struggling person to make. It's a truth that might be arrived at in time, but it might never be grasped this side of heaven. Just promise you'll never use this one as a spiritual bandage. (For more on this, read chapter 6, "Grief: Wandering through the Maze.")

*"So when are you two going to have a baby?"*
*"When are you going to make me a grandmother?"*
*"When are we going to see a little Jennifer or Steve running around?"*
What you're saying is "Hurry up! Get a move on! Keep up the pace here!" The infertile couple would love to make you a grandmother or to have little genetic carbon copies of themselves running around, but what hinders them is not of their own doing. Comments like these only exacerbate the pain.

*"I just know God is going to give you a baby soon!"*
So you've got a hot line to God that they don't? You may *think* you know, but you don't. You hope God will give your friend a baby, but you cannot definitively say so. No one on earth can. You may have felt an assurance from God as you prayed for your friend, but keep it to yourself. It just sends her on another roller-coaster ride when you throw out comments like this. A better option is to reassure her that you're going to keep praying for her during her infertility struggles.

*"Just keep praying. God will give you the desires of your heart."*
Do a little Bible study before spouting off this one. Psalm 37:4 has a preface to the part included in the above statement. It says, "Delight yourself in the Lord and he will give you the desires of your heart." Before getting the desires of our heart, we must find our delight in Him, which means that we will naturally align *our* desires with *His* desires.

**To someone who has miscarried or lost a child at birth or soon after, don't say**

*"God must have needed your baby in heaven more than we needed him here."*

This is theological heresy. God doesn't *need* babies in heaven. Plus, it makes God look like a selfish child, giving a baby to a couple and then taking it back.

*"You're young. You can always try again."*
A baby is not like a potted plant you replace when it dies in the summer heat. No future baby will ever replace the one who died. If they worked hard to get pregnant the first time, only to lose the baby, then this is a double loss for them. They have no assurance they'll be able to bring about conception again, and maybe they're not sure they can even afford it. Whether or not someone is infertile, this is a repulsive comment. Losing a baby or a child at any stage—prebirth or postbirth—is a death. That precious, unique life cannot ever be duplicated.

Treat miscarriage as the death of a child, not as the mere loss of fetal tissue. Comfort the couple by acknowledging the personhood of their unborn child. The hopes and dreams for a child's life are tied up in the expectation of an upcoming delivery, and when that child is lost through miscarriage or death, the couple feels robbed of those dreams.

*"Be glad it happened early, before you really developed a bond with the baby."*
*"At least you never held the baby; that would have made losing him so much harder."*
Guess what? They already *had* a bond with the baby, and comments like these undermined it. Holding a baby who has died is recognized by experts as a very positive way for a grieving couple to move toward closure. Among those who never got to hold their child, many would give anything to have been able to do so.

Besides, holding a baby is not when the bond begins. Feeling a baby kick inside of you is not when the bond begins. Learning you are pregnant is when the bond begins. For infertile couples, even dreaming about being pregnant is when a bond begins. Never holding their miscarried child is a heartache many couples carry forever.

## Regarding adoption, please don't say

*"After you adopt, you'll get pregnant; I know lots of people who have."*
This comment implies that adopting a child solves infertility. There's nothing about parenting an adoptive child that brings a physiological end to barrenness, causes problematic eggs to heal, or causes sperm to make it past hostile mucus. The ridiculous part of this comment is that it doesn't synchronize with earlier pieces of lousy advice. If a couple needs to "just relax" in order to get pregnant, then how in the world will they relax as new parents to an adopted child? Their lives are happily more complex with a child now, but the reality is that they're probably existing on less sleep, less sex, less quality time as a couple.

If you stop and count the number of adoptive families you've known through the years, you'll find that a much greater number of adoptive parents never bear a biological child. Of the many adoptive families I've known, only four have gone on to have biological children. It's the exception to the rule, but everyone remembers it forever—and talk about it forever, too.

*"You sure are lucky. All you had to do was adopt."*
Pregnant women are prone to complaining about weight gain, morning sickness, and a multitude of changes their bodies experience. But when a pregnant woman looks at an infertile woman and calls her *lucky* because she doesn't have fat ankles or that she doesn't get too overheated in summer, there's a need for an attitude adjustment. Infertile women long for the opportunity to feel nausea, to have food cravings, to feel a baby kick. Isn't that what you expect when you get pregnant? Isn't it normal to feel and experience all those changes?

*We had friends who experienced a difficult pregnancy and delivery. Kim was in danger of miscarriage and was limited to very restricted activity. During the delivery, she had such tearing and damage to the cervix, as well as loss of blood, that her life was in danger. After recovery, it was questionable if she would be able to conceive again. About eighteen months later, we adopted Cora, and Jim ran into*

*Kim's dad at the store. Her father said, "You and Angela sure are lucky you didn't have to go through everything Kim did. All you had to do was adopt." Even now, the statement leaves us speechless. Not to minimize their experience, but in a way, we did experience that. Angela's life was never in physical danger, but mentally and spiritually, we suffered so much as we struggled through infertility, and our final diagnosis said Angela would never conceive.*

*—Angela and Jim*

### "I'm so sorry adoption is your only option now."

I have a friend who was told this. A couple trying to get over the agony of failed fertility treatments and gearing up to adopt needs encouragement, not pity. Adoption isn't a substandard way of becoming parents.

Never offer sympathy for adoption. It's just another way God puts families together.

### "Do you know anything about the baby's real parents?"

Parents usually prefer that you not mention the child's biological parents in front of the child, especially a child who's young enough to be confused by terms and references but knows he's being talked about. One adoptive dad said he considers his children's birth parents to be more like sperm and egg donors because they are certainly not the children's *real* parents, the ones who influence them, guide them, hug them every day.

### "Who knows—you may still get pregnant and then you'll be a real mom!" or "Do you have any real children too?"

When you talk with an adoptive family, take the word *real* out of your vocabulary. By *real*, you may mean *biological*, but *real* implies authentic, the opposite of fake, genuine, the real McCoy. A man who buys an old house isn't a fake owner because he wasn't the first owner or the one who built the house. Adoptive parents aren't fake parents, and adopted kids aren't fake, either.

If you want an adoptive parent to get riled up, this is a sure way to do it. It's a deep insult to say an adoptive parent isn't a *real* parent or that his child isn't his *real* child. The parent-child bond goes far deeper than the sharing of genetic code and physical features. It's a bond formed in the heart and solidified over a million shared experiences as the years pass.

In her televised special, "Born in My Heart: A Love Story," Barbara Walters, herself an adoptive parent, interviews adoptive parents and their children. Barbara's daughter, Jackie, ha something to say about this terminology:

*"Real parent" is a really horrible label because what makes a parent is not necessarily who gives birth to you. It's the one that takes a tissue and cleans up your tears, the one that is there for the good times and the bad.*

Rosie O'Donnell, who has adopted three children (so far), was on the same TV special. She thinks it is ridiculous that people insist on labeling children as *adopted*. She told of a trip to the mall with two of her children. An older man asked if those were her adopted kids. "I started to laugh. I was like, 'They're my kids, and they were adopted, but they're not my adopted kids.' To me, it doesn't seem that way." She went on to explain that when George Burns died, a reporter described Burns's son (age 73) as "adopted." Why was it necessary to identify the son in that way?

Don't use terminology to differentiate your friends' relationship with their children as anything other than what it is: a loving, parent-child bond.

Maybe this chapter has left you a little uncomfortable, even a little frustrated. Maybe you realize you've made some of these comments to infertile friends, thinking all the while you were comforting them, encouraging them, but now you realize otherwise. Instead of beating yourself up, determine to move forward as a wiser, more sensitive friend. Listen without rushing to offer pseudo-solutions. Wade through the uncertainties with your friends instead of standing on the shore offering advice. In time, you'll see that your friends didn't need you to have the answers; they just needed you to be there for them.

# Chapter 15

# How Infertility Changes Your Perspective

*In hindsight, I wouldn't trade our experiences with infertility. Growing spiritually and being able to recognize that God is in control, even when I feel out of control, is a lesson I would have hated to miss. Many times during the process I cried, "Enough! I don't want to learn any more." But God never gave up on me. He kept working with me until I was totally dependent on Him, right where He wanted me in the first place.*  —Angela

This chapter focuses on what happens to your life perspective as a result of infertility. It explores some things you'll feel years after your infertility battles are behind you. If you're right in the middle of your infertility battles, don't read this chapter yet. Wait until you're further down the road and the raw wounds of infertility have healed some. Ideally, wait until you've become a parent or found peace with choosing to be child-free.

Why wait? Because when you're trudging through procedures, you don't need to think about this stuff; in fact, you *can't* think about it because you're in survival mode. Later on, you'll have the opportunity to look back over the Valley of Infertility and see how it has changed your life. So go on now, turn to another chapter.

### Finding flowers in the rocky valley
When poor little Joseph found himself on a slave caravan, he probably had one serious pity party all the way to Egypt. He who'd been the apple of Dad's eye was now viewed as property. In the decades that followed, he experienced unbelievable extremes: honor and trust from Potiphar, imprisonment

(thanks to Potiphar's wife), and finally, elevation to being the Pharaoh's right-hand man. We can read his entire life story in Genesis in less than an hour, tracing the hand of God through it all. But Joseph had to plod through every hour of every day of every year, eye level with his circumstances, unaware of the broader plan that God was weaving together.

If you had a bird's-eye view of your own life while you were infertile, it would have made surviving infertility so much easier to endure. You could have seen the light at the end of the tunnel. You might see why God allowed pregnancy to elude you in your younger years. You might understand why it took six failed inseminations, two surgeries, and two IVFs before you achieved pregnancy. Or maybe you'd catch a glimpse of how the failure of your first adoption attempt put you in a position to receive later the child God had for you. Or you'd comprehend why you had to experience the heart-break of infertility before it dawned on you that child-free living was is much a calling as parenthood. Your perspective makes all the difference.

But walking through the valley, you have no plateau from which to survey your surroundings. It's all you can do to keep from tripping over a boulder or getting your foot stuck in a crevice. The path in front of you occupies your full attention and concentration.

Once you resolve your infertility in some way (by solving it or resolving not to keep trying to solve it), then you begin your exit from the valley. You can, in time, look back over the terrain and see your experiences with a little more clarity. You can see that there were a few scattered flowers, tiny though they were, hidden along the way.

Maybe one flower that poked its petals from behind a rock was the friend who remained at your side through your battle. Other flowers might be the increased knowledge you have about medical matters or how to deal with insurance companies. Still another could be the empathy (as opposed to sympathy) you now share with other infertile couples who are just starting their journey, for the couple who miscarries, and for the infertile woman whose self-worth has hit bottom. The awakening (or honing) of these skills is the good you take with you from your infertility encounters.

## Another look at the family tree

One of the biggest surprises that awaited me was hidden in the branches of my family tree. While we were battling infertility, it never dawned on me to take a serious look at the plight of other females in my clan. It's certainly not the topic of discussion at Christmas get-togethers, so I never looked very far beyond my own pain.

But after we called it quits on trying to resolve infertility, I began to take a look around. I found that I was not the only one who had experienced problems with conception. Seven aunts and four cousins have had trouble conceiving and/or carrying to term. More than twice as many faced infertility as those who didn't.

When Cathy lost her first baby, Lucas, it prompted her to discover that other women in her family had a tendency to miscarry, a fact that was never talked about. If she'd known from the beginning, she would have taken precautionary measures with her first pregnancy. We learn that we have a responsibility to talk with the nieces and cousins who follow us. We need to tell our story and explain our infertility struggles, so that they won't be left in the dark to discover the problem on their own.

## Infertility can make you a better parent

I haven't found studies showing that infertile people make better parents, but I think it's safe to say it makes them more *grateful* parents. And grateful parents can be *better* parents.

Infertility forever changes your perspective on parenthood:
- You don't take for granted the ability to procreate.
- You don't assume you're "in control" of your destiny.
- You don't assume that parenthood is something you just deserve.
- You recognize parenthood as a gracious gift from God.

Never again will you come remotely close to taking your children for granted. Never again will you assume a healthy child is your inalienable right simply because you're a Christian, an American. You catch yourself before you say something offhanded about the burden of raising children:

the expense, the worry, the frustration they sometimes bring. You remember how hard you worked to get your child. Sure, they try your patience. They *are* children, after all. But in a quiet place in your heart, you remember how you ached to have a child who would one day try your patience.

Because of your battle with infertility, you're probably keenly aware of just how many people actually complain about their children, can't wait for them to be back in school each fall, long for the day that they're grown and off in college or on their own. You can't help but pity those parents. You have a perspective on life, a depth of understanding, that they have missed.

In your agonizing quest to love a child you could call your own, you learned about the bigger picture of life. You learned the value of sharing in the life of a child, whether or not it is a child who shares your genetic code. The road through the Valley of Infertility teaches you that parenthood is not for your convenience, your satisfaction, your benefit, your pleasure. Parenthood is not about being selfish; it's about giving yourself away, investing yourself in the life of the one who calls you Mom or Dad.

*I always thought I'd be a mom of more than one child, at least two, but after our IVF didn't work, I had to begin thinking of myself as the mother of an only child. I was worried that Matthew wouldn't be as comfortable with other kids, that he wouldn't have the relational skills that children with siblings have. I guess I was also concerned that he would feel cheated. But I've talked with my son, and he thinks it's no big deal that he doesn't have brothers or sisters. And I consider him to be even more of a gift now that I can't have other children. He's healthy, outgoing, and just generally a cool kid. My husband and I are able to focus on Matt's activities completely, without being split between several children's schedules. Matt knows he is so special to us. On Mother's Day he walked in while I was getting ready for church and told me, "Happy Mother's Day." I looked at him and thought, What a great kid we have! "Thank you," I said. "You're the reason I'm a mother!"* —Brenda

At a recent meeting I noticed a woman on the front row with her three well-behaved boys, ages about nine, six, and four. The leader made a comment about her new empty nest and how hard it would be to get accustomed to not having children at home. Instantly the mother of three blurted out, "You can have mine!" A few chuckles spread around the room, but I could only stare at her with a mixture of anger, disbelief, and eventually pity. Her eldest was sitting perfectly still next to her, silently taking in all she said. The other two boys were quietly playing with trucks on the floor. About a minute after she offered her smart remark, she glanced at her oldest child, looked into his eyes, and smiled warmly, as if to say, "You know I didn't really mean that." I wondered how many times he'd heard it before. I felt so sorry for those boys that they would ever have to hear a comment like that, even if it was a joke. And it took great effort for me not to corner her after the meeting and give her a quick lecture on how comments like hers can be deeply painful for grieving parents or would-be parents, not to mention what it must do to her kids.

A small number of couples discover through their infertility that they can be content without a child of their own. If parenthood is a path that calls for courage, then choosing child-free living is a road that calls for bravery. Most people don't quite know how to categorize a child-free couple. Will they be comfortable at a picnic for couples with their kids? Will they want to be around children at all? Most child-free couples enjoy and desire to be around other people's children, but they're left to prove themselves all the time as they go against the grain of a family-centered society. Child-free couples have to help others learn to be comfortable with what they believe was God's choice for their lives. Parents who were formerly infertile are most likely to understand the choice of the infertile couple to be child-free. These parents can help lead the way in showing respect, appreciation, and inclusion for child-free couples in our midst.

### Do the old feelings ever disappear?

Some of the feelings you have during your darkest days of infertility will never disappear, but they do fade. These experiences are a part of you; they're deeply ingrained. When they reemerge, their appearance can surprise you. See your response for what it is—an old wound that got bumped. Old wounds can be sensitive for years after they've healed. The scars may never completely go away, but we learn to live with them and treat them with a little extra care.

I bumped an old wound three years after we became parents. While chatting with a newly-married couple, they announced, "We're pregnant! Here's the sonogram picture!" A frightening mix of emotions swirled in my head and heart—disbelief, anger, even a bit of jealously. Hadn't I gotten beyond those feelings once we became parents?

Why do these feelings of anger or jealousy, frustration, or resentment sneak back whenever our old "infertility scars" are bumped? Because infertility deprives you of one of life's normal experiences: the predictability of bearing children. It's a loss that's never replaced in your life, even though you may become a parent. You can never go back and redo those years of your life. If your infertility was resolved through birth or adoption, then your life is full of parental responsibilities that leave little time for contemplating the pain you walked through. But when your old wound gets bumped, it's likely that some mixture of negative feelings will pop back. Don't feel guilty about it. Don't deny yourself the right to feel. Don't dwell on it intensely either. Just let it flow in and give it time to flow right back out.

I have come to grips with the fact that, yes, I am still officially infertile, and, no, I will probably never conceive before menopause erases my chances forever. I still may think *How unfair!* when a young couple marries, then gets pregnant in a snap. But I have also resolved that every now and then, when I feel a little regret pop up that we missed experiencing what comes easily for so many people, I will let the feeling rise to the surface and flow on out of me. I will let myself feel it. I won't deny it or push it back into a corner. It's a valid emotion based on what we've been through.

And always, that little speck of negativism is quickly overshadowed by Ryan's bright presence in our lives, the child who wouldn't have been here if we'd been spared the pain of infertility. It was worth it all to get Ryan.

## Minister from your own experiences
Christians exist on the mountaintop, the valley, and the

plains. Eventually, everyone sees all three locations. In traveling from one to another, we pass people on their treks to various levels. The problem is when we forget what it's like to be somewhere else.

The people on the mountaintop look out at the sky and the clouds and forget what it's like to be in the valley. Those of us on the plains go about our business every day, comfortable with where we are. Others descend to the valley and see nothing but the dry and weary land surrounding them, forgetting to look up toward the mountain for encouragement and strength to go on.

Whenever and however your infertility is resolved, don't forget the feelings that encompassed you for the season of your trial. They will uniquely qualify you to be a shoulder to lean on or a hand to lift up another.

Keep watch for opportunities to share with couples who are experiencing what you both went through. Meet them for dinner, call them, send cards and emails to them. It means more than you'll ever know; and since you've been where they are, the information will be a priceless help.

Pray for the couples you know who are attempting infertility treatments. Pray with them when you have the opportunity. Lift them up to God; plead their case before Him for His grace. You are qualified to bring them before the throne of grace in a way that others cannot. You know what you wanted others to pray for you during your journey. Pray these things for them.

*Praise be to the God and Father of our Lord Jesus Christ, the Father of compassion and the God of all comfort, who comforts us in all our troubles, so that we can comfort those in any trouble with the comfort we ourselves have received from God. For just as the sufferings of Christ flow over into our lives, so also through Christ our comfort overflows (2 Cor. 1:3–5).*

### Altered perspectives
One early spring afternoon I was puttering in the back yard when I looked over to see Ryan using his kid-sized, plastic gardening hand tools, industriously digging up a large pot of alyssum seeds. I almost called out for him to stop, but then I

caught myself. Digging up the dirt and moving small shovels-full from the pot to the ground is serious work for a three-year-old. Why should I reprimand him for exploring his world in the only way he knew how? What he was learning was much more important than protecting the contents of that planter. So I watched him, my little gardener in training.

The thought later occurred to me that in an earlier era of my life I would have rushed to stop him from disturbing the planter. On the whole, I would be doing a lot of things differently. I'd be more uptight, more exacting, more worried.

Becoming a parent at 36 has its advantages. I take life more in stride than I did at 28. I'm much more content with who I am as a woman, where we are as a couple (and now a family), and where we're going together. I've hammered out my values as my own. I've let go of a few dreams and embraced the quiet pleasures I find in reality.

It didn't seem like a loss when I shelved my goal of becoming a freelancer to learn sign language and study deaf culture so I can help prepare my little boy for a lifetime of learning. I feel like I'm refuting the old saying, "You can't have your cake and eat it too." I've done it: I had a career that gave me incredible experiences and fulfilled one part of me, and now I can fulfill another part, the part that yearned to be a stay-at-home mom. Overall, I'm a happier person. And I believe I can enjoy parenthood more now than I would have as a younger adult. My altered perspective has made all the difference.

Your perspective has been forever altered because of the struggles you survived, too. Each person's saga is unique. We were each wounded and scarred, and we are different people because of what we faced. Our perspectives have been honed by life.

For those who know Christ as Savior, we have the added benefit of knowing that our Lord was guiding us along the paths we were to take, the decisions we were to make, even (or especially) in the midst of infertility.

*"I will lead the blind by ways they have not known, along unfamiliar paths I will guide them; I will turn the darkness into light before them and make the rough places smooth. These are the things I will do; I will not forsake them"* (Isa. 42:16).

# Called first to a country, then to parenthood

When Joe and Sarah met in Asia as short-term missionaries, they knew God was calling them to each other—and to a country that had limited access to the gospel. The area where they wanted to live wasn't conducive to high-tech medical treatments.

"We began trying to get pregnant in July 1996," Sarah remembers. "The following March, I began taking Clomid, but with no results." Several months and several tests later they still had not been able to conceive. In September 1997 they went to a missionary orientation, preparing for their first term overseas. "We realized that, while we weren't overly concerned about fertility problems yet, in four years (the time of our first stateside assignment) we would be very concerned. That would be a long time to wait to have any kind of fertility testing done." So after consulting with the mission board's doctor, they began some basic testing.

Joe's reproductive outlook was fine. Sarah's doctor detected a problem that would require surgery to further diagnose. "The procedure, along with the recovery time, would delay our departure to the missions field," Sarah said. "At that point we faced a big decision. Were we going to delay going in order to continue the fertility tests or did God want us to go now? After praying about it, we felt like we really needed to go on to our assignment and trust that God would help us know how and when to follow up with testing."

In October, while still at missionary orientation, they shared their concern with three other couples. "Several nights before we left for the field, they spent some time praying for us, begging God to give us children. We felt so loved and supported as they interceded for us with such faith."

Feeling God's clear direction to proceed with their departure, Joe and Sarah left for the missions field as originally planned. "Most likely, it was in our first week there that we conceived our first child. We felt from the beginning that this was our 'Samuel.' "
The name literally means "asked or heard of God." God had heard

their prayers. "It seemed like God had chosen to close my womb for a season, and then to open it according to His own timing and plan, bringing Himself glory through this miracle," Sarah says.

Joe and Sarah serve in a country where names and their meanings are highly valued. "We take joy in sharing our testimony of Samuel and what his name means to us." When Samuel was only ten months old, Joe and Sarah found themselves expecting again, and welcomed Michael into their lives early the next year.

"When we struggle with our calling and whether God really wants us where we are, we look back at how He's blessed us in this country—first by meeting each other, and then with these boys," Beth said. "I know it's nothing that we did or didn't do that made God bless us with these children. But we're so thankful He did."

Infertility

# Glossary of Infertility Terminology

(Some portions of this glossary were compiled from the Web sites www.inciid.org and www.ivf.com.)

## Fertility Drugs and Other Medications

**Bromocriptine (Parlodel):** An oral medication used to reduce prolactin levels and the size of a pituitary tumor when present. This medication often causes dizziness and upset stomach and must be started with a small dose, which is gradually increased as needed. This medication is equally effective when the tablet is placed into the vagina.

**Buserelin:** A long-acting GnRH available in Europe as a nasal spray and used to create the pseudomenopause desirable for reducing the size and number of endometriotic lesions. It can also be used to treat fibroid tumors, premenstrual syndrome, hirsutism, ovulation induction, and for in vitro fertilization.

**Clomiphene Citrate (Clomid, Serophene):** A fertility drug that makes the brain sense a low estrogen level, stimulating ovulation through the release of gonadotropins (follicle stimulating hormones [FSH]) from the pituitary gland.

**Contraceptive, Oral:** A medication that prevents ovulation and pregnancy. Up to 3 percent of women taking the Pill will become anovulatory when they stop taking it. The regulatory effects of the Pill can also disguise symptoms of fertility problems—for example, an irregular cycle or endometriosis. May be used to control the symptoms and development of endometriosis.

**Danazol (Danocrine):** A medication used to treat endometriosis. Suppresses LH and FSH production by the pituitary and causes a state of amenorrhea, during which the endometrial implants waste away. Many women experience oily skin, acne, weight gain, abnormal hair growth, deepening of the voice, and muscle cramps with this medication.

**DES (Diethylstilbestrol):** A medication prescribed in the 1950s and 1960s to women to prevent miscarriage. Male and female fetuses exposed in utero to this drug developed numerous deformities including blockage of the vas deferens, uterine abnormalities, cervical deformities, miscarriages, and unexplained infertility. DES is no longer prescribed for this indication.

**Doxycycline:** A tetracycline derivative; an antibiotic that inhibits many of the microorganisms infecting the reproductive tract. Often used for treating ureaplasma infections. Many physicians find routine treatment with this antibiotic more cost-effective than performing multiple cultures on both the husband and wife to detect infection.

**Human Menopausal Gonadotropin (HMG), Pergonal, and Humegon:** A combination of the hormones FSH and LH, extracted from the urine of postmenopausal women. Used to induce ovulation in several fertility treatments.

**Humegon (HMG):** The luteinizing and follicle-stimulating hormones recovered from the urine of postmenopausal women. Used to stimulate multiple ovulation in some fertility treatments.

**Leuprolide Acetate (Lupron):** A drug (injected) that "turns off" the body's mechanism for producing, ripening, and releasing eggs. It is used to stop further endometriosis growth after a laparoscopy or to turn off ovulation so that it can be restarted under controlled conditions.

**Methotrexate:** A toxic anticancer drug that is an analogue of folic acid and an antimetabolite. Used as an antineoplastic agent (to attack abnormal tissue growth). Sometimes used to treat ectopic and molar pregnancies without causing major damage to the tube.

**Metrodin (Pure FSH):** An injectable form of follicle-stimulating hormone used to stimulate ovulation.

**Parlodel:** See Bromocriptine.

**Pergonal (HMG):** A medication used to replace the pituitary hormones LH and FSH. May be used to induce ovulation in women who do not respond to clomiphene citrate. Most frequently used with women who do not normally produce estrogen because of a pituitary gland or hypothalamic malfunction. May also be used with men to stimulate sperm production. (See Hyperstimulation [Ovarian Hyperstimulation Syndrome (OHSS)].)

**Repronex (HMG):** A medication used to replace the pituitary hormones LH and FSH. Similar to Humegon and Pergonal. May be used to induce ovulation in women who do not respond to clomiphene citrate. Most frequently used with women who do not normally produce estrogen because of a pituitary gland or hypothalamic malfunction. May also be used with men to stimulate sperm production.

**Serophene:** Brand name for clomiphene citrate. (See Clomid.)

## Tests, Procedures, and Specialists

**Abortion, Therapeutic:** A procedure used to terminate a pregnancy before the fetus can survive on its own.

**Alpha-fetoprotein Test (AFP):** A blood test performed to evaluate the development of the fetus and to look for fetal abnormalities.

**Andrologist:** A physician-scientist who performs laboratory evaluations of male fertility. Usually affiliated with a fertility treatment center working on in vitro fertilization.

**Artificial Insemination (AI):** The depositing of sperm in the vagina near the cervix or directly into the uterus, with the use of a syringe instead of by coitus. This technique is used to overcome sexual performance problems, to circumvent sperm-mucus interaction problems, to maximize the potential for poor semen, and for using donor sperm. (See also Artificial Insemination Donor; Artificial Insemination Homologous.)

**Artificial Insemination Donor (AID):** Artificial insemination with donor sperm. A fresh donor semen specimen or a thawed frozen specimen is injected next to the woman's cervix.

**Artificial Insemination Homologous (AIH):** Artificial insemination with the husband's sperm. The sperm may be washed and injected directly into the wife's uterus (IAIH). Often used with poor semen or to overcome sperm-mucus problems.

**Artificial Spermatocoele:** An artificial, surgically created pouch used to collect sperm from men with irreversible tubal blockage.

**Assisted Hatching (AH, AZH):** The process of thinning out the zona pellucida prior to transferring the embryo into the uterus.

**Assisted Reproductive Technology (ART):** Several procedures employed to bring about conception without sexual intercourse, including IUI, GIFT, and ZIFT.

**Basal Body Temperature (BBT):** Your body temperature when taken at its lowest point, usually in the morning before getting out of bed. Charting BBT is used to predict ovulation.

**Basal Body Temperature, Biphasic:** A basal body temperature pattern consistent with ovulation and the formation of the corpus luteum, which secretes progesterone. This hormone will elevate the basal body temperature about a half-degree during the latter half of the menstrual cycle.

**Basal Body Temperature, Monophasic:** An anovulatory basal body temperature pattern where the temperature remains relatively constant throughout the cycle.

**Beta HCG Test:** A blood test used to detect very early pregnancies and to evaluate embryonic development.

**Cauterize:** To burn tissue with electrical current (electrocautery) or with a laser. Used in surgical procedures to remove unwanted tissue such as adhesions and endometrial implants. Also used to control bleeding.

**Cervical Smear:** A sample of the cervical mucus examined microscopically to assess the presence of estrogen (ferning) and white blood cells, indicating possible infection.

**Cervical Cerclage:** A procedure in which a stitch or two is put around the cervix to prevent its opening until pregnancy is to term, then removed.

**Clomiphene Citrate Challenge Test (CCCT, CCT):** This test entails the oral administration of 100 milligrams of clomiphene citrate on menstrual cycle days five through nine. Blood levels of FSH are measured on cycle day three and again on cycle day ten. Elevated blood levels of FSH on cycle day three or cycle day ten are associated with very low occurrence of pregnancy.

**Condom Therapy:** Therapy prescribed to reduce the number of sperm antibodies in the woman by using a condom during intercourse for six months or more and by the woman refraining from all skin contact with the husband's sperm. The woman's antibody level may then fall to levels that will not adversely affect the sperm.

**Cone Biopsy:** A surgical procedure used to remove precancerous cells from the cervix. The procedure may damage the cervix and thus disrupt normal mucus production or cause an incompetent cervix, which may open prematurely during pregnancy.

**D&C (Dilation and Curettage):** A procedure used to dilate the cervical canal and scrape out the lining and contents of the uterus. The procedure can be used to diagnose or treat the cause of abnormal bleeding and to terminate an unwanted pregnancy.

**Egg Retrieval:** A procedure used to obtain eggs from ovarian follicles for use in in vitro fertilization. The procedure may be performed during laparoscopy or by using a long needle and ultrasound to locate the follicle in the ovary.

**Electroejaculation:** A controlled electric stimulation to induce ejaculation in a man with damage to the nerves that control ejaculation.

**Embryologist:** A scientist who specializes in embryo development.

**Embryo Toxicity Assay (ETA):** A combination of two procedures. The first involves maternal cell (lymphocyte) culture is aimed at stimulating the lymphocytes using components of the human embryo (trophoblast) cell line. The second is an embryo culture. These procedures are used to determine whether the patient's lymphocytes secrete anything that could be toxic to the embryo. (The test utilizes two-cell stage mouse embryos). Women who have been sensitized in the course of earlier pregnancies or in any other mode may amass an immune response against their own fetus in a later pregnancy and end up losing it (in the implantation process or later in the first trimester).

**Embryo Transfer:** Placing an egg fertilized outside the womb into a woman's uterus or fallopian tube.

**Endometrial Biopsy:** A test to check for luteal phase defect. A sample of the uterine lining is collected for microscopic analysis. The biopsy results will confirm ovulation and the proper preparation of the endometrium by estrogen and progesterone stimulation.

**Expectant Therapy (Endometriosis):** A wait-and-see approach used after laparoscopic surgery for mild endometriosis.

**Falloscopy:** The visual examination of the inside of the fallopian tube. A tiny flexible catheter is inserted into the fallopian tube through the cervical canal and uterine cavity. A small flexible fiber-optic endoscope is threaded through the catheter into the fallopian tube. A camera at the end of the falloscope transfers images of the inside of the tube to a monitor so the surgeon can thoroughly visualize and examine the inside of the tube. If problems are found, surgical repairs can be made at the same time.

**Fertility Specialist:** A physician specializing in the practice of fertility. The American Board of Obstetrics and Gynecology certifies a subspecialty for obstetricians/gynecologists who receive extra training in endocrinology (the study of hormones) and infertility.

**Fertility Treatment:** Any method or procedure used to enhance fertility or increase the likelihood of pregnancy, such as ovulation induction treatment, varicocoele repair, and microsurgery to repair damaged fallopian tubes. The goal of fertility treatment is to help couples conceive a child.

**Fertility Workup:** The initial medical examinations and tests performed to diagnose or narrow down the cause of fertility problems.

**Fertilization:** The combining of the genetic material carried by sperm and egg to create an embryo. Normally occurs inside the fallopian tube (in vivo) but may also occur in a petri dish (in vitro). (See also In Vitro Fertilization.)

**Flow Cytometric Separation (Sperm Sorting):** A process of separating sperm according to X (female) and Y (male) chromosome-bearing sperm cells for the purpose of gender selection or the prevention of gender-related diseases.

**Follicle Aspiration, Sperm Injection, and Assisted Rupture (FASIAR):** A procedure involving the use of ultrasound for guidance to remove eggs from their follicles. Sperm and eggs are mixed inside the syringe and then injected back into the patient. If the woman develops too many eggs, the physician can remove some in order to reduce the risk of multiple pregnancy.

**Frozen Embryo Transfer (FET):** A procedure where frozen embryos are thawed and then placed into the uterus.

**Gamete Intrafallopian Transfer (GIFT):** A technique that may be used in lieu of in vitro fertilization for women with patent (clear and open) tubes. After egg retrieval the eggs are mixed with the husband's sperm and then injected through the fimbria into the woman's fallopian tubes for in vivo fertilization.

**Hamster Test/Sperm Penetration Assay (SPA):** A test of the ability of sperm to penetrate a hamster egg that has been stripped of the zona pellucida (outer membrane).

**Host Uterus:** Also called a surrogate gestational mother. A couple's embryo is transferred to another woman who carries the pregnancy to term and returns the baby to the genetic parents immediately after birth.

**Hysterectomy:** The surgical removal of the uterus. May also include the removal of other reproductive structures, such as the fallopian tubes and ovaries.

**Hysterosalpingogram (HSG):** An X ray of the pelvic organs in which a radio-opaque dye has been injected through the cervix into the uterus and fallopian tubes. This test checks for malformations of the uterus and blockage of the fallopian tubes.

**Hysteroscopy:** A procedure in which the doctor checks for uterine abnormalities by inserting a fiber-optic device. Minor surgical repairs can be executed during the procedure.

**IAIH (Intrauterine Artificial Insemination Homologous):** Artificial insemination where the husband's sperm is injected directly into the uterus to avoid cervical mucus problems or to maximize the potential for poor semen. (See also Artificial Insemination.)

**Immunobead Binding Test (IBT):** Used to detect antisperm antibodies.

**Injectables/Injectable Fertility Medications:** Medications given by injection, commonly referring to ovulation induction medications such as HMG (brands Pergonal, Humegon, and Repronex), urofollitropins (brands Fertinex and Metrodin), and recombinant FSH follitropins alpha and beta (brands Follistim and Gonal-F).

**Intracytoplasmic Sperm Injection (ICSI):** A micromanipulation procedure where a single sperm is injected into the egg to enable fertilization with very low sperm counts or with nonmotile sperm.

**Intratubal Insemination (ITI):** Artificial insemination where washed sperm is deposited into the fallopian tubes. (See Artificial Insemination.)

**Intrauterine Insemination (IUI):** A relatively "low-tech" ART that deposits washed sperm directly into the uterus, bypassing cervical mucus and depositing the sperm more closely to the fallopian tubes, where fertilization occurs. Used to bypass hostile cervical mucus and to overcome sperm count and motility problems. (See Artificial Insemination.)

**Intravaginal Culture (IVC):** A procedure related to IVF where eggs and sperm are combined in a capsule and then inserted into a woman's vagina to incubate for forty-eight hours, the goal being fertilization within the woman's body. After twenty-four hours, any embryos are transferred into the uterus.

**In Vitro Fertilization (IVF):** Literally means "in glass." Fertilization takes place outside the body in a small glass dish.

**Intrauterine Device (IUD):** A device placed in the uterus to prevent pregnancy. IUD insertion has been associated with an increased incidence of infection, which may damage the fallopian tubes and is therefore not recommended for women with multiple sexual partners.

**Karyotyping:** A test performed to analyze chromosomes for the presence of genetic defects.

**Laparoscope:** A small telescope that can be inserted into a hole in the abdominal wall for viewing the internal organs; the instrument used to perform a laparoscopy. Used to diagnose and treat a number of fertility problems including endometriosis, abdominal adhesions, and polycystic ovaries. Also used in egg retrieval for in vitro fertilization.

**Laparoscopy:** Examination of the pelvic region by using a small telescope called a laparoscope.

**Laparotomy:** Major abdominal surgery where reproductive organ abnormalities can be corrected and fertility restored, such as tubal repairs and the removal of adhesions.

**Leukocyte Antibody Detection Assay (LAD):** A test that indicates a woman's physiologic response to pregnancy.

Women who test for high levels of leukocyte antibodies have a history of carrying pregnancies longer than women who exhibit low levels. Women who have low levels of leukocyte antibodies generally have had pregnancies that ended by week twelve, or their immune systems did not respond to the stimulus of pregnancy by creating blocking antibodies. Only women with low levels of LAD are candidates for immunization with their husbands' white blood cells (leukocytes), so it is recommended that this assay be done prior to initiating an immunization protocol.

**Leukocyte Immunization Therapy (LIT).** Injecting a woman with her husband's or a donor's white blood cells to increase her fetal blocking antibodies and lower her NK cells.

**Male Factor Infertility:** A general term referring to an infertility problem that resides within the male reproductive system.

**Masturbation:** A technique used to collect semen for analysis and for artificial insemination; manual stimulation of the penis leading to ejaculation.

**Micro Injection Fallopian Transfer (MIFT):** A technique similar to GIFT and FASIAR that may be used in lieu of in vitro fertilization for women with patent (clear and open) tubes. After egg retrieval the eggs are mixed with sperm and then immediately injected into the woman's fallopian tubes for in vivo fertilization. Rather than using laparoscopy, this method uses aspiration of follicles and injection into the fallopian tubes.

**Microsurgical Epididymal Sperm Aspiration (MESA):** Using microsurgery to remove sperm from the epididymis for use in IVF, often with ICSI.

**Myomectomy:** Surgery performed to remove fibroid tumors.

**Nonstimulated Oocyte Retrieval In (office) Fertilization (NORIF):** No ovulation induction hormones are used for this process (unlike SCORIF). The egg is removed by ultrasound aspiration from the ovaries. This procedure is done in the doctor's office. The egg is mixed with sperm and placed in a small plastic dish and left in the incubator for two days. The fertilized egg is then transferred to the uterus through a small plastic catheter.

**Nonsurgical Embryonic Selective Thinning (NEST):** A form

of assisted hatching using a chemical rather than scraping to thin the outer membrane of the zona pellucida.

**Nonsurgical Sperm Aspiration (NSA):** A procedure that removes sperm directly from a testicle via a tiny needle while the man is sedated. The sperm must be injected into the egg through ICSI, then implanted in the female via IVF. NSA is for men who have had vasectomies, duct obstructions, or other problems. One NSA can gather enough sperm for several ICSI/IVF procedures.

**Obstetrician/Gynecologist (Ob/Gyn):** A doctor who specializes in the diseases and the routine physical care of the reproductive system of women, including treating women through pregnancy and childbirth.

**Ovary Cryopreservation:** The process of freezing a woman's unfertilized eggs and ovarian tissue. For women delaying childbirth for an unknown period of time (such as due to chemotherapy), ovarian tissue and eggs are retrieved, frozen, and later is replaced in hopes of extending or restoring reproductive and endocrine function. The process is still "investigational" and is not covered by insurance plans.

**Ovarian Drilling:** During a laparoscopy, an electrosurgery needle is used to burn ten to twelve small holes into each ovary. This procedure may help reduce androgen levels and restore cycles in women with polycystic ovaries.

**Ovarian Wedge Resection:** Surgical removal of a pie-shaped wedge of a polycystic ovary in order to help ovulation.

**Ovulation Induction:** Medical treatment performed to initiate ovulation. (See also Clomiphene Citrate; Pergonal.)

**Paternal Leukocyte Immunization (PLI):** Injecting a woman with her husband's (or male partner's) white blood cells to increase her fetal blocking antibodies and lower her NK cells.

**Penile Implant:** A device surgically inserted into the penis to provide rigidity for intercourse. Used to treat impotence.

**Percutaneous Epididymal Sperm Aspiration (PESA):** A small needle is passed directly into the head of the epididymis and fluid is aspirated. Any sperm found are used in IVF with ICSI.

**Perinatologist:** A doctor specializing in treating the fetus/baby and mother during pregnancy, labor, and delivery, particularly when the mother and/or baby are at a high risk for complications.

**Postcoital Test (PCT):** A microscopic examination of the cervical mucus best performed twelve or more hours after intercourse to determine compatibility between the woman's mucus and the man's semen; a test used to detect sperm-mucus interaction problems, the presence of sperm antibodies, and the quality of the cervical mucus.

**Preimplantation Genetic Testing:** A genetic disease management process currently being developed, in which IVF is used to produce early embryos which are biopsied, sometimes as early as the four-cell stage. The embryos undergo testing to see if they carry specific genetic diseases, such as Huntington's disease. Only embryos free of the disease would be implanted in the female, thus assuring that future generations will not carry on that particular disease.

**Progesterone Withdrawal:** A diagnostic procedure used to analyze menstrual irregularity and amenorrhea; uterine "bleeding" that occurs within two weeks after taking progesterone; a procedure used to demonstrate the presence or absence of estrogen and to demonstrate the ability of the uterus and reproductive tract to "bleed." Prior to ovulation induction therapy, progesterone withdrawal may be used to induce a menstrual period.

**Reproductive Endocrinologist (RE):** A medical specialty combining obstetrics and gynecology with endocrinology to treat reproductive disorders.

**Reproductive Immunologist (RI):** A medical specialty combining obstetrics and gynecology with immunology to treat reproductive disorders that are related to immune problems.

**Reproductive Surgeon:** An ob/gyn or urologist who specializes in the surgical correction of anatomical disorders that affect reproductive function.

**Salpingectomy:** Surgical removal of the fallopian tube.

**Salpingolysis:** Surgery performed to remove adhesions that restrict the movement and function of reproductive organs.

**Salpingostomy/Fimbrioplasty:** Surgical repair made to the fallopian tubes; a procedure used to open the fimbria.

**Selective Reduction (SR):** A controversial procedure in multiple pregnancies that terminates (aborts) one or more embryos so that the other embryos have an increased chance of survival.

**Semen Analysis:** A laboratory test used to assess semen quality: sperm quantity, concentration, morphology (form), and motility. Also measures semen (fluid) volume and whether or not white blood cells are present, indicating an infection.

**Sonogram (Ultrasound):** Use of high-frequency sound waves for creating an image of internal body parts. Used to detect and count follicle growth (and disappearance) in many fertility treatments. Also used to detect and monitor pregnancy.

**Sperm Bank:** A place where sperm are kept frozen in liquid nitrogen for later use in artificial insemination.

**Sperm Washing:** A laboratory technique for separating sperm from semen, and separating motile sperm from nonmotile sperm, for use in assisted reproduction.

**Split Ejaculate:** A method used to concentrate the sperm for insemination; separating the semen into two portions: the first portion of the ejaculate is rich in sperm, and the second portion contains mostly seminal fluid.

**Stimulated Cycle Oocyte Retrieval In (office) Fertilization (SCORIF):** The woman's ovaries are stimulated with medications such as HMG or pure FSH. The eggs are removed by ultrasound aspiration from the ovaries. This procedure is done in the doctor's office. The eggs are mixed with sperm and placed in a small plastic dish and left in the incubator for two days. The fertilized eggs are then transferred to the uterus through a small plastic catheter.

**Superovulation:** Stimulation of multiple ovulation with fertility drugs; also known as controlled ovarian hyperstimulation (COH).

**Surrogate Mother:** A woman who is artificially inseminated and carries to term a baby who will be raised by his or her genetic father and his partner.

**Testicular Biopsy:** A minor surgical procedure used to take a small sample of testicular tissue for microscopic examination, used to diagnose male fertility problems when no other means is available (the biopsy procedure itself may cause testicular damage).

**Testicular Sperm Aspiration (TESA):** A needle biopsy of the testicle used to obtain small amounts of sperm. A small incision is made in the scrotal skin and a spring-loaded needle is fired through the testicle. Usually does not result in enough sperm to freeze for later use.

**Testicular Sperm Extraction (TESE):** An open biopsy where a small piece of testicular tissue is removed through a skin incision. The tissue is placed in culture media and separated into tiny pieces. Sperm are released from within the seminiferous tubules where they are produced and are then extracted from the surrounding testicular tissue. This procedure can be done using local anesthetic of IV sedation. It is possible to get enough sperm to freeze for future use.

**Transuterine Fallopian Transfer (TUFT):** The placement of an embryo inside the fallopian tube after IVF. The transfer is made by threading a tube through the cervical canal and uterus and depositing the embryo into the fallopian tube. The process is meant to mimic the natural process of a fertilized embryo traveling down the tube and implanting in the uterus.

**Tubal Embryo Transfer (TET):** The placement of an embryo inside the fallopian tube after in vitro fertilization. The process is meant to mimic the natural process of a fertilized embryo traveling down the tube and implanting in the uterus.

**Tubal Ligation:** Surgical sterilization of a woman by obstructing or tying the fallopian tubes.

**Tubocornual Anastomosis:** Surgery performed to remove a blocked portion of the fallopian tube and to reconnect the tube to the uterus. Tubouterine implantation may also be performed to remove fallopian tube blockage near the uterus and reimplant the tube in the uterus.

**Tubotubal Anastomosis:** Surgery performed to remove a diseased portion of the fallopian tube and reconnect the two ends; sterilization reversal.

**Ultrasound:** A test used instead of X-rays to visualize the reproductive organs; for example, to monitor follicular development and to examine the tubes and uterus. The instrument works by bouncing sound waves off the organs. A picture displayed on a TV screen shows the internal organs.

**Urologist:** A physician specializing in the genitourinary tract.

**Vasectomy:** The accidental or elective surgical separation of the vasa deferentia; a procedure used for birth control.

**Zygote Intrafallopian Transfer (ZIFT):** An ART in which eggs are removed from a woman's ovaries, fertilized with the man's sperm in a lab dish, and the resulting embryos transferred into the woman's fallopian tubes during a minor surgical procedure.

# For More Information

## Internet Resources

**RESOLVE, The National Infertility Association,** at
www.resolve.org
Helpful articles about coping with infertility, coping with the
holidays, advice, and information about new treatments.
Check to see if a local RESOLVE chapter meets near you.
(RESOLVE; 1310 Broadway; Somerville, MA 02144;
[617] 623-0744)

**American Society for Reproductive Medicine (ASRM),** at
www.asrm.com
Loaded with factual information that can be read online, some
of which can be downloaded free. (ASRM; 1209 Montgomery
Highway; Birmingham, AL 35216-2809; [205] 978-5000)

**The InterNational Council on Infertility Information
Dissemination (INCIID),** at www.inciid.org
Provides an extensive list of fact sheets, a glossary, and an
amazing list of answers under "General Infertility FAQ."
(INCIID; P. O. Box 6836; Arlington, VA 22206; [703] 379-9178)

**National Adoption Information Clearinghouse,** at
www.calib.com/naic
Offers a long list of free documents to answer questions about
adoption. (The best online resource for adoption information I
have located.) (NAIC; 330 C Street, SW; Washington, DC
20447; [703] 352-3488 or 1-888-251-0075; fax: [703] 385-3206)

**National Council for Adoption,** at www.ncfa-usa.org
Provides general information on adoption as well as guide-
lines for deciding to adopt and taking the first steps. (NCFA;

1930 17th Street NW; Washington, DC 20009-6207; [202] 328-1200; fax: [202] 332-0935)

**Holt International Children's Services,** at www.holtintl.org
This adoption agency's site lists many of the companies who offer adoption benefits plans. Go to their Web site and search "Benefits." (Holt International Children's Services; P. O. Box 2880; Eugene, OR 97402 [541] 687-2202; fax: [541] 683-6175)

**National Adoption Center,** at www.adopt.org
Provides information on a variety of topics, plus a photo gallery of children waiting to be adopted. (National Adoption Center; 1500 Walnut Street, Suite 701; Philadelphia, PA 19102; 1-800-862-3678)

**Tapestry Books,** at www.tapestrybooks.com
This company focuses solely on listing books on the topics of adoption and infertility. An especially unique collection is the books for children who are adopted. (Tapestry Books; P. O. Box 359; Ringoes, NJ 08551; 1-800-765-2367)

**American Academy of Adoption Attorney,** at www.adoption-attorneys.org
This national association lists attorneys who practice in the field of adoption law. Their Web site lists members' addresses and phone numbers. (AAAA; P. O. Box 33053; Washington, DC 20033; [202] 832-2222)

**Mommies Enduring Neonatal Death,** at www.mend.org
MEND is a Christian, not-for-profit corporation reaches out to those who have lost a child due to miscarriage, stillbirth, or early infant death and offers ways to share experiences and information through support groups, a bimonthly newsletter, and a Web site.

**Crown Financial Ministries,** at www.crown.org
This ministry offers financial planning resources from a Christian perspective. A few examples of resources are *The Complete Financial Guide for Young Couples, Discovering God's Way of Handling Money* Course Workbook, *Money in Marriage.*

**The Nurturing Network,** at www.nurturingnetwork.org
This nonprofit organization was launched by a woman who
experienced miscarriage and wanted to find a way to offer
help to women with unwanted pregnancies who were choosing abortion because of their desperate situations. TNN's
advocacy on behalf of birth mothers offers them respect,
resources, and nurturing carried out by a grassroots organization of over 30,000 volunteers.

## Books

*How We Grieve: Relearning the World,* by Thomas Attig (New
York: Oxford University Press, 1996)

*When Empty Arms Become a Heavy Burden,* by Sandra Glahn
and William Cutrer, M.D. (Nashville: Broadman and Holman,
1997)

*All of the Women of the Bible,* by Edith Deen (San Francisco:
HarperSanFrancisco, 1983).

*Surviving Pregnancy Loss,* by Rochelle Friedman, M.D., and
Bonnie Gradstein (Boston: Little, Brown and Company), 1982

*Men & Grief: A Guide for Men Surviving the Death of a Loved
One; A Resource for Caregivers and Mental Health Professionals,*
by Carol Staudacher (Oakland, Calif.: New Harbinger, 1991)

*Tracks of a Fellow Struggler,* by John Claypool (New Orleans:
Insight Press, Inc., 1995)

*Disappointment with God: Three Questions No One Asks Aloud,*
by Philip Yancey (Grand Rapids: Zondervan, 1988)

*Childless Is Not Less,* by Vicky Love (Minneapolis: Bethany
House, 1984). This book is currently out of print, but may be
available in used bookstores, libraries, or via interlibrary loan.

*Sweet Grapes: How to Stop Being Infertile and Start Living Again,* by Jean Carter, M.D., and Michael Carter, Ph.D. (Indianapolis: Perspectives Press, 1989)

## Magazines

**Adoptive Families Magazine,**
at www.adoptivefamiliesmagazine.com
For subscription prices and ordering information,
call 1-800-372-3300.

**Ferti Magazine,** at www.ferti.net

## Television Specials/Movies Worth Watching

**"Born in My Heart: A Love Story,"** aired April 20, 2001. This Barbara Walters special is a warm, honest look at adoption from domestic and international perspectives. Barbara's only child gives her first public interview about being adopted. (ABCNewsStore.com)

*Baby Dance,* 1998, produced by Jodie Foster. This movie portrays the tension between a poor couple who decides to place their fifth child for adoption and an infertile couple trying to locate an adopted child. The plot accurately shows financial, emotional, legal, and relational issues. (available on video)